HUMANITY 0 – CORONAVIRUS 1

What Next?

HUMANITY 0 – CORONAVIRUS 1

What Next?

R. Peprah-Gyamfi

Published by Perseverance Books
www.peprah-gyamfi.com
email: info@peprah-gyamfi.com

© Copyright R. Peprah-Gyamfi 2020

HUMANITY 0 – CORONAVIRUS 1
WHAT NEXT?

ISBN: 978-1-913285-07-4
eISBN: 978-1-913285-08-1

Contents

Introduction: A wrestling encounter gone horribly
wrong 1

**Part one   Reminiscing on the last quarter of
a decade gone too soon 5**

Chapter 1A   Divided opinions in an imperfect world 7

Chapter 1B   The seven continents of a single planet   11

Chapter 1C   Three worlds in one 19

Chapter 1D   One nation, one people, one destiny..........20

Chapter 1E   Those who consider themselves too
intelligent and honest to join the
political circus 21

Chapter 1F   When arch-enemies meet for good-
natured banter..24

Chapter 1G   26 billionaires, 3.8 billion humans and
a common planet......................................27

Chapter 1H   Starvation in the midst of plenty 29

Chapter 1I   Advances without end on an imperfect
planet..30

Chapter 1J   Greta Thurnberg here we come!................33

Chapter 1K   Superstars, celebrities and role models
of the world 34

Chapter 1L   Space tourism on the horizon!...................36

Chapter 1M Great expectations for a new decade...........38

Part two **A daredevil leap into the future** **41**

Chapter 2A Mission impossible – "expedition humanity" 43

Chapter 2B A missed opportunity with consequences 46

Chapter 2C Happy New Year 2020! 48

Chapter 2D Replication en masse in hijacked cells 49

Chapter 2E How could King Corona have anticipated this?! 52

Chapter 2F When speed is of the essence.................... 54

Part three **Time for soul-searching** **59**

Introductory note 61

Chapter 3A The powers that be giving Corona a free ride... 63

Chapter 3B How the behaviour of the general public facilitated the spread of Corona....... 69

Chapter 3C Indirect human factors facilitating the spread of Corona 74

Part four **Corona is here to stay** **77**

Chapter 4A The gist of a 100-page report.................... 79

Chapter 4B The humble contributions of a concerned citizen.................................... 81

Chapter 4C Gearing ourselves for the inevitable.......... 91

Appendix 96

My heartfelt condolences and deepest sympathy goes to all who have lost family members and loved ones to the awful Covid-19 pandemic raging around the globe. I am also deeply saddened by the heart-breaking situations of those who have lost their livelihoods, their jobs, their savings, their investments due to the direct and indirect effects of this horrible plague.

As we mourn our dead and continue to grapple with the effects and repercussions of the still ravaging pandemic, it is my hope that humanity will at long last realise the need to work together as an entity to tackle the plague with our concerted rather than divided efforts, so as to enable us get on top of the problem and, in so doing, contribute towards the return of normalcy on earth, to the way of life we were accustomed to prior to the emergence of the impudent novel Coronavirus, aka SARS-CoV-2, in our midst.

Introduction:
A wrestling encounter
gone horribly wrong

As in the case of several of her age in her village, the birthday of my mother, who departed this life in July 1994, was not recorded. Not only was her date of birth unregistered, she also did not enjoy the privilege of formal education.

In the matter of formal education, her children had an advantage over her – Ghana's first president, Kwame Nkrumah, who led the then Gold Coast into independence, introduced free and compulsory education into the newly-independent country, renamed Ghana.

The "young academics" in her home eventually set out to resolve the mystery surrounding her date of birth.

The only source in our small settlement we could resort to was an elderly man in our midst. Affectionately called Uncle Tom by all, he was unique in not a few respects. He was the only individual in the community who benefited from formal education, his parents having paid for him to attend school at a settlement far away from ours (there was no school in the village).

In the course of his life, Uncle Tom turned himself into an unofficial "registry" of births and deaths in the community. Using his meagre resources, he acquired a notebook and a pen, and began dutifully to record the dates of births and deaths of every single individual of the community – something which the state had not thought necessary to do!

According to our beloved Uncle Tom, he experienced the awful influenza pandemic that raged through the world in 1918–19 as a teenager. He spoke tearfully about the suffering and deaths he witnessed. He also spoke of reports that reached the village of deaths in the big towns, including the capital Accra. In Accra, he told us, it appeared as if there were many more deaths than the living to dispose of the bodies.

Though he had at that point in time not assumed his unofficial office as the registrar of births and deaths in the settlement, he made it known to us that our mother was born not long after the horrendous scourge had left the devasted earth populace in peace. The information of our beloved "civil servant" led us to settle on 1920 as the probable year of birth of the indispensable anchor of our family.

Was it due to the link established between the 1918 pandemic and mother's age? I cannot say for sure. The fact remains that in the later years I developed interest in the topic, which led me to research it further. In particular, I was desirous of establishing how a problem that is said to have first affected US military on their home soil managed to spread to our small village – at a time when global air travel was nothing more than a future dream?

In the event, I learnt that in all the pandemic led to the deaths of about 2% of the African population. It is said to have entered the continent by way of various sea ports. In the matter of West Africa, I established that the virus first arrived in Freetown in the capital of the English colony of Sierra Leone aboard a Royal Navy warship that had arrived from England. The virus had raged on the ship during its journey from England to the West African port. By the time the ship docked there on 14 August 1918, 124 of its crew had fallen ill from the virus.

Owing probably to the reluctance of the port authorities to disrupt naval operations, no strict quarantine measure were followed. Instead workers and medical staff were permitted to board as well as leave the ship. Within days of the arrival of the ship, a large proportion of the sailors as well as the staff at the port had become infected. From Freetown the virus ravaged across the entire West African region and beyond.

Though there have been numerous epidemics as well as a few pandemics since then, never did I imagine I would live to witness a pandemic on the scale of the 1918–19 plague.

Like most other residents of a world that has become closely interconnected, I learnt about the coronavirus outbreak in China in the course of December 2019.

Much as I pitied the residents of Wuhan in particular who bore the brunt of the initial outbreak, and the residents of China in general, the problem appeared to be too far away to bother me personally.

Then came January 2020, and the first case was reported in Europe – the continent of my residence. At that stage, I realised that it was no more a Chinese problem but rather a global one, which needed a co-ordinated global approach to the matter – I was to be disappointed.

Many global leaders, instead of listening to scientific advice, took their own course. Many of them began to resort to the term "war". "We are at war; I am a war-time president" one global leader was quoted as saying. On one occasion, as I watched a global leader on TV talk of war between humanity and coronavirus, an idea flashed through my mind. "Okay, if everyone is talking of war, then you just position yourself as a war-time correspondent, reporting from the battlefield!"

Since it was the army from Coronaland that first attacked humanity I needed to find a motive for their action. Initially, I thought of corona attacking us for being too noisy and causing too much pollution!

As the death toll from the pandemic grew higher with each passing day, with TV pictures from Italy depicting lines of military vehicles transporting the dead to their graves, I decided, for the sake of the dead and their mourning relatives, to soften my approach on the matter, in order not to be accused of being insensitive to the suffering of others.

Still, I could not avoid the issue of "motive". What led the newcomers from Coronaland to venture into the human realm to cause such havoc? In the end I settled on the fact that the microbes wanted to extend their realm of existence.

King Corona told a meeting of the Council of Elders he had summoned to announce his plans to send expeditioners to the human kingdom:

> "We have all along been living with horse bats. As you will agree with me, we have all along had a very cordial relationship with them over the last several hundred years.
> Whenever we accompany the horse bats on their nightly excursions to the settlements of humanity, we see such beautiful streets, wonderful cars, bright streets. Much as we have devel-

oped very cordial relationships with the horse bats, in my view, we need to expand our realm. Nobody knows tomorrow. Anything could indeed happen tomorrow to wipe out the entire population of our hosts – that would signify the end of our race as well. To avert that situation happening, I have thought it wise we expand our realm into the human kingdom as well."

Thus, in the same way that humans are exploring space for signs of life, which could perhaps allow some of our contemporaries to settle there in future, King Corona decided to send expeditioners to explore the possibility of settling with humans.

Having settled on the motive for their incursion into the human kingdom, I pondered over the title for my book project.

Many will agree with me that, apart from the human death and suffering, the newcomers have caused extensive disruption to various aspects of life on earth. It is thus not unfair to state that the match – a wrestling match perhaps – has so far gone against humanity. Initially, I thought of a thrashing, humiliating scoreline of 10–0 in favour of the guests. In the end, I decided on a face-saving score of 1–0.

The cut-off date for my report is 31 July 2020.

It is superfluous to say that the match is not over yet. I cannot rule out producing a second report in the near future. Hopefully, humanity will by then have learnt from their mistakes and turned the tide in their favour. Until then, I wish everyone joy in reading the account of this field reporter.

Part one
Reminiscing on the last quarter
of a decade gone too soon

Chapter 1A

Divided opinions
in an imperfect world

The first decade of the twenty-first century, also regarded as the third millennium, was gradually drawing to a close. Humankind, which has been on planet earth for God knows exactly how long, were going about their lives as usual.

Though life on planet earth is not heavenly, humanity seem to have come to terms with the imperfection.

Residents get up in the morning to engage in their various daily routines – care for their children; attend schools, colleges, universities; go to work etc. At the end of their daily activities they return home – if they have a place they call home, for indeed some among them have no fixed abode and are forced to dwell on the streets – to rest, to wake up the next morning, to begin yet another day. Thus, life goes on, in an imperfect world.

From time to time disasters, both man made and natural, rock parts of the planet. Thanks to modern forms of communication, TV for example, images of the catastrophes, are beamed worldwide, into the living rooms, offices, pubs and restaurants etc. of the inhabitants. For a while, the sympathies of common humanity are aroused; many respond to the calls for help with generous donations. For a while, the tragedy dominates the headlines. But soon the story of the human misery gradually disappears from the public domain – till the next disaster strikes.

One thing peculiar about humanity is that it seems to lack consensus on pretty much everything. Indeed, apart from five areas pertaining to their life on earth where there is general consensus, their opinions, views, belief, outlook and what have you digress on virtually everything else!

I want to touch briefly on the five areas where there is universal agreement within humanity on the core issues.

Firstly, it is fact, which none of them can deny, that every one of them arrived on planet earth naked.

Next is the manner of their departure from earth – just as they arrived here unclothed, they also depart nude and helpless.

The next three issues over which the usually divided humanity generally agree upon pertain to what is universally regarded as the three essentials of life – air, water and food.

Indeed air, to be specific oxygen, is so vital for life – deprived of it, human life ceases within a matter of minutes.

I have just touched upon the five areas where there is general agreement among humans.

There ends the cordiality; beyond that humanity is in dispute over every area of their existence. I will touch on a few such controversies in due course.

Unfortunately, some of these disagreements not seldom lead to conflict, not only between individuals, but between nations.

It is just astonishing, for at the end of the day they are all visitors to the planet, yet too often hefty disagreements ensue between individual humans as well as nations over pieces of land and property! Such disputes sometimes leads to stabbings, shootings, massacres, to substantial loss of live.

I better leave mysterious humanity alone, otherwise I am in danger of going haywire and veering off course!

One of the most enduring points of contention among humans revolves around how they got to planet earth to begin with. One would have expected a broad consensus on such a fundamental question of where they came from. How did the universe come into being and, most importantly, how did they themselves get here. But that is not the case.

Concerning the issues of how they got here, there are broadly three schools of thought on the issue.

The first group credits a supernatural being, Almighty God, with the creation of the universe, and all that it contains, including themselves.

The second group does not believe in a Creator God. Their view is that the universes came about out of chance and that life also evolved out of mere chance.

Between the two schools of thought are a group that believes that lesser gods and not an Almighty God are behind the universe and all the different forms of life it contains.

It is beyond the realm of this book to delve into the details of all the beliefs, assumptions and conjectures held by humans in regard to the origin of the universe and life on earth.

Concerning human beings themselves, they share several features and characteristics. To name just a few – each human possesses a head, a nose, a pair of eyes, ears, arms and legs etc.

One would have thought they would concentrate on the myriads of things they share in common and pay little importance to the slight differences in their external features, such as the colour of the hair, eye, skin etc.

Ach! humanity, aka homo sapiens! Dwelling on their differences appears to be the driving forces, the fuel needed to propel them through the universe!

A notable example revolves around the issue of the colour of their skin. It is an undeniable fact that not all human beings are endowed with the same colour of skin. Instead, there are various shades of colour ranging from the darkest brown to the very palest skin hue.

As far as the author of this lines is concerned, it makes good sense that that is the case. One can imagine how monotonous it would be for a world to be populated by around 7.8 billion residents all endowed not only with the same skin colour, but also exactly the same colour of hair and eyes.

Conversely, how glorious is the present rainbow society of mankind, featuring various types of skin hue ringing from darkest brown to pale.

But complex humanity!

What was meant to bring diversity into the room, a myriad mixture of colours making a beautiful mix, has become such a huge point of contention, leading to conflicts too numerous to count!

It might as well require a gathering of the most scholastic, brilliant and outstanding minds, to deliberate, philosophise, delve into some of the inherent traits of humanity that has contributed to such a state of affairs.

I better let the matter to rest and carry on with the task I have set myself, before I run out of precious time.

In any case, as at the fourth quarter of 2019, humanity had not completely ridden itself of the prejudices, scorn, disdain etc. they hold for each other over many issues, including that pertaining to the type of skin colour one is endowed with.

Chapter 1B
The seven continents
of a single planet

Though someone viewing their planet, planet earth, from space would tend to see one entity, humankind for its part over the years agreed to partition it into continents. Though there are variations in the definition of continents, the most widely accepted definition is a large, continuous, discrete mass of land, ideally separated by an expanse of water.

There are in all seven continents. They are named alphabetically as follows – Africa, Antarctica, Asia, Australia and Oceania, Europe, North America, South America.

I want to take a short overview of the continents. I want to make it clear from the very onset that I am doing so in alphabetical order. Anyone not familiar with humanity will wonder why I have gone to lengths to stress that fact. Humanity! They are so sensitive – some might otherwise accuse me of favouritism, bias, discrimination and what have you. So here we go.

Africa

Africa is the world's second-largest and second-most populous continent, occupying an area of about 11.7 million square miles and boasting a population of around 1.3 billion inhabitants.

Africa could as well be described as a continent of paradoxes and contradictions – very wealthy in minerals and natural resources, and yet home to some of the most deprived residents on earth. Indeed, whereas the great majority of the populace were facing abject poverty, the 52 heads of state of the continent were doing very well, enjoying a good life in their opulent presidential palaces. Which brings to my mind a quote from George Orwell's Animal Farm: "All animals are equal, but some animals are more equal than others."

As if they harbour a sense of disdain towards their own healthcare system, the leaders have cultivated a habit of boarding their presidential jets and heading outside of Africa, to far distant lands, to seek treatment for even mild conditions that could be dealt with by their own doctors.

The common man and woman on the streets of Africa can aptly be compared to a person caught between a rock and a hard place – they are not only exploited by their leaders, the whole international economic system appears to be working against them, a situation that has led many a well-wisher of the continent to give up in despair.

Indeed owing to factors, too numerous to count, as the continent was heading for the second decade of the twenty-first century only a few optimists still held any prospect of Africa coming out of the doldrums anytime soon.

Antarctica

Antarctica is the continent occupying the southern-most tip of the planet. It is an icy expanse that stretches to cover more than 5.5 million square miles, temperatures are consistently below zero throughout a majority of the year. Due to the fact that it remains extremely cold for most of the year, it is almost uninhabitable.

One would have thought humanity would leave the vast icy expanse to rest in peace, to declare it a natural reserve out of bounds from any kind of human activity. But no! As at the time period under consideration, there were around 30 different countries operating 80 research stations on the vast expanses of the "no man's land!".

Asia

Asia is not only the largest continent on earth, occupying an area of approximately 17,212,000 square miles, it also boasts a population of around 4.6 billion inhabitants.

I want to take a closer look at a few of the countries in Asia.

China is the country boasting the highest population on earth. Over the last several years, it has been transformed from a deprived country to become one of the leading global economies.

India, China's neighbour to the west, is usually labelled the world's largest democracy. Whether the deprived of places like Mumbai, Calcutta and New Delhi would rather prefer a guarantee of a regular supply of their daily basic necessities – food, clothing and shelter– to their country's reputation of being the largest democracy on earth, is a question that I would love to put to those faced with abject poverty in the populous country.

I nearly forgot Japan. Though not as populous as the her two Asian neighbours, she is a mighty global player economically, boasting, as at the fourth quarter of 2019, the world's third largest economy, on the basis of her gross domestic product (GDP).

Australia and Oceania

The two most important countries of Australia and Oceania are Australia and New Zealand. During the period under consideration, Australia was visited by a huge raging fire that persisted throughout the fourth quarter of 2019. Though the country is prone to such fires, this particular one was generally regarded as beyond the ordinary.

Europe

After the turbulent years of the twentieth century, the century that saw Europe as the main battleground for two horrible global conflicts, conflicts that initially began on European soils and later spread to the rest of the world, leading them to gain the accolade "World", instead of European wars, Europe was flourishing. One could well refer to a bonus resulting from 75 years of peace.

For a while Europe was partitioned by the virtual iron curtain dividing Communist Eastern Europe from the capitalist West.

Hardly anything on planet earth lasts for ever. That is exactly what happened on 9 November 1989 when the concrete wall dividing West Berlin from East Berlin was torn down by citizens of the eastern side of the divided city. With the fall of the Berlin wall, not only was divided

Germany reunited, the whole of Europe, thankfully, was also reunited.

Before I end my brief excursion of the European continent, I want to take a quick look at the state of the European Union, the EU.

On 25 March 1957 the Treaty of Rome, which was meant to end the bloody conflicts that had been the lot of Europe over the years, was signed between Belgium, France, Italy, Luxemburg, the Netherlands and West Germany. It came into force on 1 January 1958.

As at the beginning of the fourth quarter of 2019, it had 28 members. In the middle of the period under consideration, namely on 12 December, something significant happened. One of its members, the United Kingdom took a step that would see the number reducing to 27. On that day, a general election was held that ended with a clear victory for the Conservative party, which had vowed to implement the results of the Brexit referendum that had been held three years before. Thus, barring the unexpected happening, come 31 January, the EU was set to lose one of its main members.

Before, I move on, I will briefly touch on Russia, which, geographically, forms part of both Europe and Asia. Russia used to be part of the Soviet Union, which ceased to exist on 31 December 1991. I personally thought that after the fall of the Berlin wall and the unification of Germany and Europe at large, there would be more cordial relations between Russia and the rest of Europe. For a while that seemed to be the case. But, typical humanity! The cordial relationship did not prevail for very long. "Poor farmer's son from rural Ghana, you better not get yourself involved in the explosive sphere of complex geopolitical politics" I hear someone whisper into my ear. Good advice good fellow! These days one has to be careful when it comes to such matters, otherwise one runs the danger something happening to cause the big-mouthed individual to just vanish from the surface of the earth!

Still, I dare just quickly pass a short comment on the matter.

Was Russia perhaps aggrieved by the fact that all the former members of the Communist Bloc that formed the Warsaw Pact chose to join their former arch enemy, NATO, instead of at least keeping neutral? Looking at it from a human perspective, my gut instinct tells me that could well be the case.

The Russians are humans after, not angels. Let us just come to consider the matter on a personal level. Assuming you have a business partner. You wake up one day to find the individual has left your company to team up with your competitor. Human as you are, for a while you will feel aggrieved, won't you?

Matters have of late become even more complicated with various Western leaders accusing Russia of interfering in their democratic elections. "If indeed the Russians did meddle in their elections, then it serves them right. They have since time immemorial meddled in the affairs of us, their former colonies!" said a school mate in Accra in an email, who had just got wind of what I had just written. Please, don't query me on the matter, for it did not originate from me!

In any case, as at the fourth quarter of 2019, Europe, though the smallest continent on earth, was doing quite well, with her two voices on the UN Security Council and looking forward to 2020.

North America

North America is made up of two countries, the USA and Canada. Canada to the north is the second largest country on earth. Despite its huge size, it boasts a population of just 38 million. It has one of the youngest among the world leaders. At the end of the fourth quarter of 2019, it was at peace with itself.

That takes me to Canada's mighty neighbour to the south, the United States of America. While making up just 4% of the world population, according to IMF figures for 2020 it boasts 23.6% of the world's GDP.

One can understand why it is still regarded as the world's economic powerhouse, a superpower not only in military terms, but also in economic terms.

Its huge wealth has made its currency, the dollar, the world's leading currency.

The saying has it that wealth attracts wealth. Indeed, due to its abundant wealth, I get the impression that practically everything that is produced on the globe heads for that country!

Whether made in China, the EU or South America – the US market serves as an attraction. The saying "the rich will get richer" is aptly demonstrated here, for even though some residents live in absolute scarcity and lack the very barest needed to lead a life expected of humans, they are overlooked by the global producers of wealth. Instead goods are shipped to a US market already saturated with its abundant supply of goods.

It is not all a blessing though. Indeed, not only "good" items – the likes of food medicine, clothing – reach there, but also the "bad" ones as well – cocaine, heroin, amphetamine etc.

The abundance of goods of all sorts including food – all types of food – appears to have its downside. Is the sight of abundance of food wherever one turns serving as a temptation too strong to resist for a good proportion of the population? In any case that is the impression I gain when I watch TV footages showing people walking the streets of the mighty nation. In such moments, I do say to myself: my goodness, that country has without doubt an obesity problem!

For several years, the US played not only the role generally regarded as the "world's policeman", it also generally played open door politics with the rest of the world.

That changed with the arrival of Mr President "America First" on the world political scene in January 2017. The moment he took the oath of office, he declared to the whole world: "Ladies and gentlemen, take it from me – with immediate effect it is going to be 'America First!'"

It was not mere words. Indeed ever since then, he has vigorously pursued his "America First" policy.

Thus as at the fourth quarter of 2019, it could be safely said that Uncle Sam was virtually in self-isolation. It is astonishing how unsettling things can be in an ever-changing, unstable world! One day America is playing the global policeman, doing all it can to bring order into a confused world, the next day, going into a complete lockdown, self-imposed quarantine!

Not only has the ex-world policeman gone into self-seclusion, it is also planning a huge, impregnable concrete wall, which will dwarf the ancient wall of China in magnitude, vastness, impregnability, dimensions and what have you.

Concerning the relationship of the US with its two direct neighbours, north and south, it is not free from occasional irritations. This has become notable since President "America First " came to power in 2017. Of course, I cannot ever imagine any period in time when such irritations get out of control, leading to armed conflict with one of them, or both at the same time!

Well, as at the fourth quarter of 2019, Uncle Sam was at peace with itself. Those who are politically inclined were looking forward to the presidential elections in November 2020.

South America

As at the last quarter of the first decade of the twenty-first century South America, referred to by many as Latin America, was generally at peace with itself.

Mexico, one of the main countries, was not in an enviable position. By virtue of sharing frontier to its northern superpower neighbour, it has become the battleground for various drug lords seeking to gain a share of what appears to be the lucrative drug market of its northern neighbour. Besides, the frontier has been drawn into the never-ending confrontation between immigrants hoping to make it to the US on the one hand and the border guards seeking to prevent them from crossing into the "paradise on earth" on the other.

I nearly forgot Brazil, one of the main countries of the continent aside from Mexico and Argentina. The name Brazil has become almost synonymous with football. I heard two blokes engaged in a heated argument the other day as to which one of the following is more accurate: "when football dies Brazil dies" or "when Brazil dies football dies"! They stopped me on the street and asked my opinion on the matter, to which I replied, they better contact the "football god" Pele himself.

Dwelling on football, nearly led me to forget about another important Brazilian icon – namely the Amazon forest! 2019 was not a particularly good year for the Amazon forest. For reasons that are beyond the remit of this discourse, unusually high numbers of bush fires raged in the huge forest for much of the year. Whereas the flamboyant president of the country regarded the matter as an internal issue, several other countries, especially those in the Western world thought otherwise.

"Your country cannot, dare not lay sole claim on the Amazon forest. Are you not aware, that forests serves as the lungs of our common planet?" they argued. The president reacted angrily to the intervention, accusing the Western powers of unwanted interference in the internal affairs of a sovereign country.

The author of these lines whilst saddened by the destruction of the forests was also surprised to hear the rest of the world, in particular the Western leaders, all of a sudden speaking of the lungs of a common planet. Common planet? Really strange – for, as I will touch upon shortly, it is generally held by all and sundry that there are currently at least three different worlds!

Chapter 1C
Three worlds in one

One would have thought that humanity would be satisfied with the partitioning of the planet solely on the basis of the seven continents. But no!

Several years ago, someone came up with the concept of classification, not based on geography, but rather on wealth and influence.

In the end, the originally solitary world became three different worlds! The first of the three was assigned to the rich, industrialised countries. With wealth comes power; the countries of the first world thus have considerable influence in world affairs.

The second world was designated to countries of the Communist Bloc in Eastern Europe. Although the Communist Bloc has broken, the former countries of the alliance have still retained their designation as second-world countries.

Last, but not the least, is the third world, which consists of developing countries in Africa, South America and Asia.

Chapter 1D

One nation, one people, one destiny

Mankind! They have also gone further to divide planet earth into different sovereign states.

Several centuries ago, the idea of the creation of nations began. Language might have played a role. There are several languages on earth. How do you communicate with someone you cannot understand? So, logically, those speaking the same language began to gather together. Another factor – conquest and colonialism – contributed to the development. So mankind divided into nations and states. As at the end of the fourth quarter of the twenty-first century there are generally considered to be 195 countries.

In order to cement their partition into states, and also to prevent criminals, the beggars, the poor, the dying etc, from fleeing from one part of the world to their countries, nations came up with borders. There are several forms of borders. There are those that are virtually non-existent, as pertains with the borders between most European countries. At the other extreme are national borders that are not only portioned by way of concrete walls, barbed wire, other forms of physical demarcation etc., but are additionally secured by way of landmines, armed guards, and other security devices etc. – for example the border separating the two Koreas.

Chapter 1E

Those who consider themselves too intelligent and honest to join the political circus

In order to create order in their respective countries, in order not to allow things to descend into anarchy, nations came up with the idea of national governments, with authority to execute order and discipline in their respective countries. Thus each country has a form of government.

Some countries are ruled by dictators. The words of such dictators are final and whoever dares challenge them risks death.

So far, the form of government that has gained widespread acceptance is what is termed a "democratic" form of government or "democracy". I will touch on the matter of democracy briefly.

For the system to function, elections are held at regular intervals, usually every four to five years, with the goal of electing representative to represent the various constituencies in parliament. In an ideal world, one would expect only the most upright, most intelligent, honest, incorruptible, men and women of very high standing and calling, to be elected –the best of the best, the almost infallible, the best brains around, chosen to deliberate on the problems facing their respective societies. Well, in the imperfect world of mankind, that hardly or rarely happens.

The most intelligent among the many have different interests and priorities. Indeed some of the best brains in town may prefer to become scientists in their effort to solve some of the problems brought about by virtue of the their existence in an imperfect world with imperfect behaviour – pollution for example.

Others may decide to devote their energies towards finding cures to some of the diseases afflicting mankind – cancer for example – and developing vaccines/antidotes to fight some of the diseases caused by germs.

Not only the intelligent among them may turn their back on the art of governance; the very honest, the men and women of integrity, those of high calling, may also decide not to become politically engaged. The honest men and women of character may be repelled by an aspect of the game of politics that, while not completely fulfilling the designation "lying", is not very far from it.

But it may well be the case that a certain proportion, even if very small, of those classified as intelligent, honest, forthright, individuals of the highest integrity, despite the flaws of the "game of politics", may still want to become involved – only to realize just at the onset they do not possess enough *quids* (English), *Knete* (German), *kudi* (my native Twi) to enable them to pay their way through the gruesome, tiresome, time-consuming campaigning carnival. They have hardly joined the campaign carrousel before they give up in utter despair!

Partly as a result of the above factors, humanity often ends up being ruled by not the very smart, but rather populist and wealthy individuals, individual who are very economic with the truth.

Thus as they were heading towards the year 2020, one could say, with all good conscience, that those selected in various countries to their respective parliaments could not be described as the best boys and girls in town.

One peculiar feature of homo sapiens is that, sadly, they appear incapable of resolving problems through negotiations. Thus conflicts that could be settled by way of mouth soon degenerate into war. Or is it because the leaders who send the soldiers into conflict do so from the comforts of their offices, far removed from the battlefield? Oh the poor soldiers! So often they are sent to the frontline by leaders who, probably out of arrogance, are unable to exercise humility in their negotiations with each other. Here too, I do not want to delve into details.

During the first half of the twentieth century, humankind was engaged in two bloody world wars. To prevent a third catastrophe happening, they came up with the idea of the United Nations. Though it is not a perfect organisation, it has at least managed to keep a semblance of peace on an imperfect planet earth.

Every year in September the UN General Assembly takes place at the headquarters of the organisation in New York. Almost every leader of the 195 member countries attends – the most brilliant, the medium brilliant, the brilliant, the less brilliant, the .... I dare not go further due to concerns I could be accused of disrespect for the his/her excellencies – leaders duly sworn into the highest offices of their respective countries! Every year they gather and report to the whole world as to how gloriously things are moving on in their very corner of our magnificent world.

The last gathering took place only a few days prior to the arrival of the fourth quarter of 2019. The participants, having enjoyed the cosy life of New York, the city that is affectionately dubbed "the city that never sleeps", were looking forward to the next meeting in the year 2020.

Chapter 1F

When arch-enemies meet
for good-natured banter

Though they are settled on a common planet, which they did not create themselves, several factors – suspicion, national pride, feeling of insecurity etc. – has led to distrust among nations.

Though as already mentioned, they have the UN club, still nations have found it necessary to set up defence forces to defend their respective countries from attack from both real and perceived threats.

I don't have the figures, but everyone agrees that on the whole nations spend trillions of dollars with the goal of defending their respective countries from each other – a situation that leads a layman in matters of national defence strategies such as me to ask myself: how come nations don't just sign non-aggression pacts with each other?

Let us take some of the trouble spots of the world. How about South and North Korea signing a non-aggression pact with each other, a pact that does not exist only on paper but will be observed to the very letter?

How about all the countries of the Middle East signing non-aggression pact with each other – Israel with the Palestinians, Israel with Turkey, Israel with Iran, Iran with Afghanistan, and so on, until all the countries of the region have signed non-aggression pacts with each other.

That would not be the end of the matter. To celebrate the peace, they would also hold a big festival of sports and games – hockey, football, whatever each of them is interested in. Finally, there could be a big party of reconciliation to enjoy Mediterranean cuisine and other dishes.

Just imagine it! the Israeli president sitting side by side with his Middle Eastern neighbours around a dinner table, enjoying some good meals and chatting about some of the day-to-day challenges we all face as human beings– agonising toothaches, pulsating migraines, persistent arthritis pain, unending family feuds etc.

What about the president of the US inviting the presidents of China and Russian to an informal meeting at a bar somewhere in downtown Washington? Away from the public glare, and in jovial exchanges centred on some of the silly antics they did as boys with the aim of catching the attention of the girls they so much adored, they could perhaps receive a burst of insight concerning the need for nations to strive to live together in peace for their mutual benefit.

That sudden burst of inspiration could well lead them to launch a global non-aggression initiative with the goal of getting each country on planet earth to sign a non-aggression pact with every other country – a commitment/protocol that would not exist only on paper, but will be honoured to the very letter by each signatory!

Having signed up to such historic declaration, the trillions of dollars that would otherwise have been spent annually on arms could be used to build decent accommodation for the poor of places like Calcutta, Lagos, Sao Paulo, who are forced to live in dilapidated structures under conditions that, without doubt, are not fit for human habitation.

Someone reading this has just emailed me to tell me this is just a utopian way of looking at things that can never happen. Well, I mentioned earlier that this is an idea from a layman in matters of warfare. It is very sad, really. If we could just sit down and realise that, at the end of the day, this place does not belong to anyone, so we had better learn to live in peace.

In any case, at the last quarter of 2019, distrust among nations was as prevalent as it has always been.

Earlier on, I pointed out there is universal agreement concerning the three basic necessities of life – air, water and food.

Air is available to everyone, though there are big differences in quality across the world.

Though from time to time water becomes scarce in some parts of the globe, especially in the Middle East and parts of Africa, one can fairly say that both are generally available.

The matter is not clear cut when it comes to food. Whereas all experts agree that at the fourth quarter of 2019, there was enough food on earth to go round – that based on the stock of food on planet earth no one needs to die of starvation – sadly not everyone is able to meet their minimum daily food requirement. Several factors – distribution, affordability, conflict etc. – account for this absurd situation.

Chapter 1G

26 billionaires, 3.8 billion humans
and a common planet

As with all other issues pertaining to humanity, there is divided opinion as to how wealth should be distributed.

Basically there are two schools of thought. One is that wealth should not be private. In other words, the state should have complete control of ownership and distribute the wealth which, by definition under this system, belongs to the whole of society according to the needs of the citizens. That is communism.

Whereas it sound reasonable on the surface, it has a weakness – it fails to take into account the basically egotistic human nature. Human beings are so egotistical and self-seeking, selfish, greedy – everyone wanting to keep things for themselves. So it collapsed.

At the other end of the scale is capitalism, where investment in and ownership of the means of production, distribution and exchange of wealth is made and maintained chiefly by private individuals or corporations.

It is generally accepted that human beings tend to be selfish. It has led to a situation where, currently, wealth is concentrated in the hands of only a small fraction of the human race.

According to an Oxfam International report published recently, the combined fortunes of the world's 26 richest individuals reached $1.4 trillion in 2018 – the same amount as the total wealth of the 3.8 billion poorest people. A situation where only 1% of the world's population controls half of the entire wealth of the world is, in my opinion, untenable!

Wealth is not only unequally divided among individual living in a specific country, it is also unevenly divided among nations. Several factors, beyond the remit of this discussion, account for this. Some countries just have the fortune of having huge reserves of minerals and oil beneath them, helping them to become rich. That is not a guarantee of wealth though. Indeed there are countries that are sitting on abundant natural reserves in which their citizens are nevertheless impoverished due to many factors – poor governance, economic mismanagement, corruption, etc. God knows whether they can ever come out of their poverty.

It was not a perfect world, but at least people were getting on with their lives. They were getting married and reproducing. Despite the eternal tension that has always existed between the two genders, they have continued to co-operate in the providential plan to use both as agents in the multiplication of humanity, to prevent them from going into extinction – something that the other creatures they share the planet with might not be particularly unhappy with. Ach, the prospect of getting rid of their troublesome partners!

Talking of wealth and wealth distribution leads me to touch briefly on the trade in stocks. As at the end of the fourth quarter of 2019, life was going on as usual in the stock exchange arena. Despite the volatile nature and uncertainties of the international financial market, human-kind seemed to have accepted it as an inevitable part of life, a testi-mony to how imperfect life on earth is.

For example, in October 1929, a stock market crash wiped out mil-lions of investors, leading to the Great Depression, the worst economic downturn in the history of the industrialised world. It would last for almost a decade – yet, astonishingly, at least from the point of view of a layman, the stock markets still hold centre stage in world commerce.

Apart from the turbulence that has become part and parcel of the trade, no one reckoned with anything unusual, come 2020.

Chapter 1H

Starvation in the midst of plenty

As at the fourth quarter of the , there were about 7.8 billion humans populating the planet. Awesome! If one sits down to consider the amount of food needed every day to feed 7.8 billion hungry mouths – awesome!

Actually, they have enough food to go round, but for several reasons – economics, poor transport networks linking the place of production and the hungry mouth needing to be fed – a considerable proportion of the world population struggles to find their daily bread.

Chapter 1I

Advances without end
on an imperfect planet

In the area of medicine, great strides have been made over the last few centuries. As at the fourth quarter of 2019, doctors are able to put patients asleep and perform complicated surgeries. That was not always the case. Indeed, up until the discovery of ether anaesthesia in 1846, all surgeries – minor and major – were performed on the still conscious patient. One could imagine the pain such patients had to endure.

As they looked towards the advent of 2020, the surgical world could celebrate some of the achievements of the last several years – the transplant of hearts, kidneys and lungs. We are able to perform surgery on foetuses.

As they try to operate on diseased organs, surgeons inadvertently introduce germs into the bodies of their patients. Today, many such infections are taken care of by antibiotics; that was not always the case. Indeed, up until the discovery of penicillin in 1928 by Alexander Fleming, even the least form of infection could end up being fatal.

Great strides have also been made in the area of medical diagnostics. As humankind headed towards the new decade in 2020, sophisticated devices and gadgets – dialysis machines, magnetic resonance, heart–Lung bypass machines, CT scanners, robots and lasers – were being employed in most places in the diagnosis and treatment of various kinds of diseases.

It must be pointed out here that, just as in the distribution of wealth, in the area of medical care, not every citizen on the planet was benefitting from the great advances of the last several years.

Indeed, whereas citizens in some parts of the world do enjoy what can be described as extreme medical care, where residents enjoy excellent medical care from the cradle to the grave, those living in other parts of the same planet have access to little or no medical care on getting unwell.

The author of these lines could indeed bear testimony to the inequalities touched upon. As he made his advent to planet earth, his big head got stuck in the birth canal of his poor mum! With no professional midwife, let alone a doctor , to skilfully intervene to bring an end to the precarious situation, the labouring and the poor "traveller" were left to themselves and providence. That he is able to report about the matter several decades on is a testimony to the favour Heaven has and continues to show in his life. Through the invincible hand of providence, your truly managed to emerge from the perilous situation unscathed, to the delight of all the participants.

Whereas those who live on the sunny side of the awful divide can reckon with a stay of anywhere between 80 and 90 years on earth, those not so blessed can call themselves lucky if they manage to make it past 60 years.

Though everyone is aware of the imbalances, as at the fourth quarter of 2019, residents of the world seem to have grown accustomed to the situation and were not expecting any radical changes in the years ahead.

At the end of the first decade of the twenty-first century, mankind had made great advances in the area of science and technology. Of particular note is the area of information technology –some call it the IT revolution. Thanks to the breathtaking advances in that sphere, as humanity headed for 2020, the talk was about the whole world having developed into a kind of global village. Indeed the moment something happened in one corner of the globe, it soon became a global event, thanks to social media platforms like Twitter, Facebook, YouTube.

Technological advancement led mankind over the years to think even bigger, to make ever bigger plans. Even though they are confronted with myriads of problems on earth, they saw the advancement in technology as an opportunity to venture into space – an area of the universe that had fascinated some members of the human race for years. Finally after years of endeavour, in 1961, the Russians sent mankind's first manned flight into space– carrying a Russian by the name of Yuri Gagarin.

The Russian feat triggered a kind of competition, between the USSR and the US. In 1969, the American succeeded in sending the first human to the moon. Since then they have carried out several missions into space. In 1971 humankind built their first space station.

As if the peaceful exploration of space was not enough, towards the end of the fourth quarter of 2019, on 21 December 2019 to be precise, the US president, amid a big fanfare, launched a "space force" to display US superiority in space. The new military unit of the so-called remaining world superpower is said to have an annual budget of $738 billion!

Chapter 1J
Greta Thurnberg here we come!

Human activity leads to pollution of the atmosphere. Over the last several years, though activists had been highlighting the problem, not much attention has been paid to the issue by the policy makers.

Everything changed with the arrival of a Swedish teenage girl by the name of Greta Thunberg. For reasons that the author of these lines cannot exactly pinpoint, she manged to galvanise global attention to the problem in a manner no single individual before had manged to do!

Though her actions have helped invigorate, to arouse, to stir debate on the issues, to the several issues confronting humanity, it has been difficult to find a consensus. Whereas some of the adult population and the overwhelming proportion of the youth are for the taking of immediate measures towards climate change, part of the adult population, for various reasons – money no doubt is one – have been reluctant to commit fully to the cause.

As they stood at the end of the first decade of the twenty-first century, the general thinking was that the climate change activists were gradually winning the debate. Would the pendulum continue to swing in their favour in the coming years? Of course, ordinary humans that they are, none of them could predict what would happen in the years ahead.

Chapter 1K

Superstars, celebrities and role models of the world

All work and no play makes jack a dull boy, so the saying goes. So mankind has come up with ways of entertaining and engaging themselves – in sports, music, films etc.

Talking of films, a huge industry has developed around it globally. Once a year, the top performers assemble in the Mecca of their privileged club, Hollywood, in what has been named the Academy Awards or Oscars. During the event, the aura and the atmosphere of which many, including the author of these lines, have great difficulty finding appropriate adjectives to describe – awards in various categories are bestowed on the performers, some of whom appears in outfits that seemed to have been produced on a planet different from our own.

One cannot touch on the entertainment industry without touching on fashion – indeed both departments of human endeavour work hand in hand, for indeed it is fashion that dresses the stars and superstars of the film world. As at the last quarter of 2019, a huge fashion industry had established itself on earth. At regular intervals fashion shows are organised. For someone the likes of the author, who grew up in the deprived environment of an impoverished village, I begin to wonder if they live on a different planet. In any case I hardly come across anyone on the street wearing some of the extravagant outfits that are displayed on the catwalks. Well, those versed in the business tell me that indeed people do wear them.

Humanity does not only resort to films to entertain themselves. They have over the years developed myriads of sporting and recreational activities.

Among the popular sports of humanity are football(known as soccer in some parts), tennis, basketball, golf etc.

Long, long ago humanity engaged in such activities only as a way of entertaining themselves and breaking the boredom. Well, along the way, others decided to make a profession out of what used to be just a pastime. The spectators enjoying watching such games were asked to contribute a bit by way of entry tickets to help support the players and their families – which of course is a legitimate demand – life on earth cannot go on without paying bills; indeed paying bills has become one of the most important activities of human life.

In due course, humanity invented mass media agents such as radio, newspapers, TV, internet etc. These media helped to transmit events to a mass audience, millions and sometimes even billions of viewers across the globe. The more the global audience, the more cash flew into the accounts of the media giants.

"We are not stupid!" the players, athletes, performers of the various sporting events declared. We deserve a fair share. Initially the organisers of the events were reluctant to play ball. Eventually they gave in to the demands of the athletes.

That led to the coining of the term "sports millionaires". The sports millionaires do not only have access to abundant wealth, they are also designated the title of celebrities and are looked upon as role models by the rest of society.

On the matter of celebrities, stars, superstars etc.: some of them get paid millions for doing practically nothing whilst others, for example teachers, carers, nurses perform tedious work and get paid get paid next to nothing. Although there is a general consensus that this is a state of affairs that calls for reform, everyone seem to have accepted it.

Chapter 1L

Space tourism on the horizon!

Tourism had become big business by the fourth quarter of 2019. Why not? The planet is made for all of us, so there is nothing wrong with others travelling around to explore other places.

As in many aspects of life on earth, however, it seems to be something for the people of the first world. Much as a little farmer's son from a place in the remote Congo forest would like to travel to a place like Disneyland to enjoy the fascinating events and shows, how can they afford the issue of their travel documents. Even if they managed to pay for the passports, how could they convince the US consulate, or in case they wanted to visit Disney Europe the French consulate, to issue them with a visa?

I can see in my mind's eye such an individual appearing there with his parents in tattered clothes and telling the consulate officer – please, we are here to apply for a visa to your country.

In the best-case scenario the officials may tell them they might have lost their way; in the worst-case scenario, they could ask them to visit the next psychiatric hospital for a check to determine their sanity!

On the contrary, a child of his age born to US American parents could just travel at will with his parent to have an adventure in the Congo forest if they so wished – without even the need to call on their embassy in their country.

The fact that some could travel easily to destinations of their choice and others cannot has led to terms such as slum tourism, passport apartheid etc.

It must be stressed that travel around their globe is not restricted to land travel. Travel on water has been one of the oldest from of movement from one place to the other. Very long ago, it was by way of simple rafts, boats, ships etc. Travel on water was used mainly for the transportation of goods. But of late another aspect has been added to it, namely cruise ships – a kind of hotel on the waves. They are becoming ever more luxurious. Those who can afford it just leave the trouble of land behind them and venture unto the sea. One might describe it as luxury on the high seas.

Travel on land we can; travel on water we can; but what about travel in the air?

"Yes, we can!" The Wright brothers – Orville and Wilbur – declared in their workshop in Dayton, Ohio, USA. Soon, they went about to try to realise their ambition. After many failed attempts to lift off the ground, on 17 December 1903, the yearning of humanity to conquer the air was rewarded when the Wright brothers undertook the first ever engine-powered flight. With the invention of the airplane began travel around the globe, which brought a boost in tourism.

I nearly left out space travel!

Well as at the end of the fourth quarter of 2019, space travel has been limited to the experts. Going forward, there are many efforts to extend the tourist industry into space.

Chapter 1M

Great expectations for a new decade

As we approached the end of the second decade of the twenty-first century, the shops in the rich Western industrial countries were as usual filled with all sorts of items. Notable at this period of year were items meant for the Christmas season. Christmas was around the corner.

Talking of Christmas, it was originally instituted by the Christian world to celebrate the birth of Jesus, who His follows regard as the saviour of the world. Though according to the narrations he was actually not born at that time of year, it has been a tradition to celebrate the occasion on that day.

Though a good proportion of the population of Europe, the continent that used to be the stronghold of Christianity, do not want to have much to do with the faith, for various reasons they look forward with joy to the occasion. Retailers and other business ventures are delighted with the shopping boom associated with it. Even before the last quarter had been ushered in, the shops were getting themselves in good shape for the expected burst of commercial activity.

Other are happy at the opportunity to meet family members who they have not seen for a while. For others it is party time, a time for merrymaking

The new year 2020 was expected to usher in some important anniversaries, significant events milestones etc. 8 May 2020 was to mark the 75th anniversary of the end of World War II. Huge events were planned, in several parts of Europe to mark Victory in Europe Day, VE Day, to celebrate the victory of the Allies over Nazi Germany.

In the area of sports, fans were looking forward to the usual annual series of events in tennis, golf, motor sports, American Football, the

English Premier league etc. Besides the routine events, two major events were scheduled for the year.

Ardent football fans, such as the author, was looking forward to the sixteenth European Football Championship. Dubbed Euro 2020, it was scheduled to take place from 12 June to 12 July 2020. The 2020 event was to be unique in one respect. Instead of being hosted by a single country, or in rare instances by two countries, this one was to be played in several countries around the continent – a one-off event to celebrate the sixtieth anniversary of the competition.

Then there was the Tokyo Olympics – the mammoth quadrennial global event scheduled to start on 24 July and end on 9 August. Athletes the world over had been spending months, if not years, painstakingly preparing for the event.

This author was also keenly looking forward to the event. Over a 16-day period humankind, at least the sports lovers amongst them, would either directly or through the media enjoy numerous sporting events. For a little over two weeks, sports lovers would be privileged to enjoy the events and, if only for a short while, put aside some of the worries, cares and troubles of everyday life.

At the end of the fourth quarter of 2019 life on earth was proceeding quite peacefully.

That does not mean there was heaven on earth. Throughout history, there have been conflicts, misunderstandings between individuals, groups, organisations, nations on earth. etc. One of the conflicts zones that had experience recurring flare ups, the Middle East, was relatively quiet. The war in Syria had been raging for over eight years. Though there had been long periods of quiet on the battlefields lately, from time to time flare-ups were reported. Then there is the perennial tension along the frontiers of North and South Korea. At the unification of Germany in 1990, one would have thought both countries would follow suit –as at the end of 2019, there was no sign of that happening any time soon.

Despites the squabbles between individuals and nations, squabbles petty and major, despite the huge gulf between the rich and the poor, despite wars and conflicts simmering in various parts of the globe, as the year 2019 was drawing to a close, it was fair to say that humanity was settled pretty peacefully on planet earth.

Part two
A daredevil leap into the future

Chapter 2A

Mission impossible –
"expedition humanity"

Unbeknown to humanity, as people were going about their lives and looking forward to the advent of the year 2020, a meeting that would turn out to have huge repercussion on their way of life on earth was taking place in Coronaland.

On 22 October 2019, King Corona summoned the council of elders to his residence. Apart from two officials who excused themselves by virtue of ill health, every one of the nine-member powerful council of elders attended.

After everyone had taken their seat, the king began to address them:

"We have all along been living with horse bats. As you will agree with me, we have all along had a very cordial relationships with them over the last several hundred years.

Whenever we accompany the horse bats on their nightly excursions to the settlement of humanity, we see such beautiful streets, wonderful cars, bright streets. Much as we have developed very cordial relationships with the horse bats, in my view we need to expand our realm. Nobody knows tomorrow. Anything could indeed happen tomorrow to wipe out the entire population of our hosts – that would signify the end of our race as well.

To avert that situation, I have thought it wise we expand our realm into the human kingdom as well.

Towards that goal, I have come up with a plan, Expedition

Humanity, to send a team of seven expeditioners – men and women of strength, stamina and endurance – to go and dwell with humanity for a while and ascertain whether they could serve as a second suitable host for our population, apart from the horse bats.

The team will report back on a regular basis concerning their experience with humanity, at the latest in six months, and, based on their report, I will make a final decision as to the way forward."

In the Kingdom of Coronaland the word of the king is final. In the end, therefore, it was agreed to dispatch the seven as proposed by the sovereign.

The seven would seize the best possible opportunity to launch themselves into the body of the humans during one of their trips with the horse bats into the human kingdom.

After undergoing a few days of fitness training, on 11 November 2019, the seven Corona expeditioners set out on their mission, all of them stuck onto the under surface of a horse bat on a nightly adventure to homo sapiens country.

The expedition did not go as smoothy as they had envisaged. To their initial disappointment the horse bat fell unwell midway through the journey and decided to return home. Fortunately, just about the time the horse bat made an emergency landing with the goal of resting a while to garner energy for the return journey, a pangolin emerged from the woods. The scaly land-based mammal exchanged cordial greetings with its compatriot with the unique capability of flying. In the event, the horse bat informed the newcomer concerning the seven expedition-ers he had planned to carry to the human kingdom and how they were utterly devasted at the prospect of having to abandon their mission.

"You don't have to be disheartened!" the pangolin assured the seven eager adventurers. "I am heading for the outskirts of a human community in search of food. I am happy to conceal you in my body."

"That is very kind of you" the seven expeditioners replied, as if with a single voice.

Excited at the favourable turn of events, the seven adventurers left the body of the horse bat and settled in the pangolin. Soon the ways of the pangolin and the Corona expeditioners on the one side and that of the horse bat on the other separated.

The pangolin had travelled barely half an hour when he was seized upon by a hunter. The pangolin was not killed; rather it was caged and sent to a huge wildlife market in a city which, as the newcomers from Coronaland later discovered, happened to be Wuhan in China. In view of the large number of humans frequently in the area, the expeditioners from Cornoaland had little difficulty in catapulting themselves one after the other into seven different humans – three male and four female.

Chapter 2B
A missed opportunity
with consequences

Starting from 15 November, that is just a few days after the news arrivals from Coronaland had made their incursion into the bodies of the seven humans, some of those affected, who happened to be residents of Wuhan in the Hubei province of China, began to feel irritations to their body – mainly in the form of coughing and sneezing. What initially began as banal flu-like symptoms began to look more serious, with those affected developing persistent coughs and significant breathing problems.

Nothing to worry about, the affected encouraged themselves. Seasonal flu can sometimes give rise to the symptoms they were presenting. Meanwhile some had sought medical help. The doctors, just like their patients, initially thought they were dealing with some of the known complications of respiratory viral infection such as bacterial secondary infection (more of which later).

As far as the newcomers from Corona country were concerned; it was life as usual. They did not notice any difference than with the horse bats but for the fact that their new hosts provided them much more space to grow and multiply. Indeed, whereas in the horse bats they could multiply only a few hundred times, in the case of humans they could do so exponentially.

Towards the middle of December, anxiety was growing within the medical community of Wuhan and its surroundings. As the number of patients who were coming into admission with symptoms of the mysterious pneumonia-like respiratory diseases that was not responding to any antibiotics grew, doctors and other healthcare personnel became astonished. One of the leading doctors is quoted as saying " Damn it! I have been working for the last 20 years but I have not come across anything like this!"

Test results initially confirmed it was SARs, a respiratory disease epidemic that broke out in the Guangdong province of southern China in 2002–03, and which resulted in more than 8,000 cases in 26 countries.

Doctors in the Wuhan Hospital where the cases of the mysterious "pneumonia of unknown origin" were being treated shared the news with their colleagues in the Chinese social media chat room We Chat. Soon news of the outbreak of "pneumonia of unknown origin" started circulating more widely.

One of those doctors who started spreading the news was Dr Li Wenliang, an eye specialist who worked at the Wuhan Hospital. Instead of the local authorities taking the matter seriously, they sought instead to suppress the truth. In the event Dr Li Wenliang, who later became a victim of the disease, was contacted by the police and warned to stop "making false comments".

Chapter 2C
Happy New Year 2020!

New Year's Eve is usually party time on planet earth; 31 December 2019 was no different. Throughout the day, all across the globe, intense preparation were made towards the huge parties, events and celebrations that were to get underway a few hours prior to midnight, in anticipation of the arrival of the new year 2020.

By virtue of its westernmost location on the planet, Auckland in New Zealand, traditionally, was the first major city on earth to welcome the new year. As the clocks struck midnight, amid fanfare and a great deal of extravaganza, the multitude that had gathered in various locations in the city cracked open bottles of champagne and cheerfully toasted the New Year. For several minutes thereafter huge fireworks lit the night sky of the metropolitan city on the North Island of New Zealand.

How could any of the humans making merry foresee the significant disruptions to their daily living that the new year had in store for them?!

The celebrations moved on to Melbourne and Sydney in Australia. In the course of time, the New Year 2020 arrived in Tokyo, Beijing, Moscow, Berlin, Paris, London, New Yok and, last but not least, San Francisco.

Chapter 2D

Replication en masse in hijacked cells

The newcomers from Coronaland had, in the meantime, begun to replicate en masse in the bodies of their human hosts. Through various activities of their original human hosts – spitting, coughing, sneezing– their offspring were passed on easily to other human residents.

Nine days into the new year, 2020, several weeks after they first launched themselves into humans, the Chinese authorities finally came to terms with the new reality. They were dealing with organisms that, while having similarities to the SARS of 2002, were slightly different in their structure. The humans finally decided to name them as 2019-nCoV.

That brought home to them memories of a problem they had encountered in 2003 with the SARs outbreak. Once bitten twice shy. Acting on the wisdom of that saying, they took urgent steps to help contain the problem. On 23 January 2020, the authorities placed Wuhan, a city with a population of 11 million people, under total lockdown.

Meanwhile their hospitals were no longer able to cope with the influx of patients. What was to be done?

Well they did something which even their worst of enemies could not help but applauding. They built a 1000-bed emergency medical facility in just 10 days to meet the increased demand to treat emergency Covid-19 patients.

Despite their divisions, a so-called revolution in information technology had virtually created a global village. In other words, what happens in one corner of the planet is easily transmitted to other parts of the planet. Thus, within days, the news of the new mysterious disease and the problem affecting their compatriots in China entered the international public domain.

It was a pitiful to watch the misery that had befallen the residents of Wuhan.

Despite their initial attempt at downplaying the extent of the problem, on realising what was the cause of the condition, the Chinese authorities did what they could to inform the rest of the world about the emergence of the new intruders to planet earth.

Having in the meantime encoded the genetic make-up of the newcomers, the Chinese authorities shared the information with the rest of the world so as to, among other things, develop a suitable test for their presence in the human body and, most importantly, develop the necessary antidote against them.

In the meantime the death-toll in the human population continued to rise, sending panic among the population.

The new arrivals from Coronaland were astonished, dumfounded, at the unexpected turn of events. They had over the last several centuries co-existed peacefully with horses bats without causing them harm, without causing them any adverse effects.

They had fed on them, replicated themselves in their body, had accompanied them in their daily activities, flying around, hunting for insects – all the activities associated with their daily lives. That had led them to assume that relocating to the human community would not cause their new hosts any harm, that things would proceed as smoothly as in the case of their long-term compatriots.

How could the simple and unsophisticated beings know that the body of the horse bats had adapted themselves, had developed something known as permanent immunity, to their presence, a fact that had permitted the bats to tolerate them without any adverse effects to their bodies.

Was it due to human's inherent trait to be selfish, a trait that had led them to develop the inclination to keep everything to themselves and not want to share with anyone else? Was it just because their bodies, caught on the backfoot, were so surprised at the unannounced intrusion of the foreigners into their bodies that they began to behave in an irrational manner? One can only speculate!

The fact remains that, instead of repulsing the visitors, directing the counterattack against the invaders, their defence systems reacted in a haphazard manner, to the extent they began targeting themselves, inflicting damage to themselves! That unfortunately turned out to be the case with a good proportion of the human hosts.

Indeed, no longer had the newcomers settled in the bodies of their human hosts than some of the humans began to feel unwell. Some, after the initial bodily reaction, recovered. In some cases, the body system of their human hosts reacted just as in the case of the horses bats – they displayed virtually no symptoms of the disease. For a good proportion of humans however, especially the elderly and those burdened with various preconditions, it led to significant/severe deterioration in health, including, in some cases, their demise.

At the end of the first week of their mission, the newcomers relayed the unexpected developments to their king. In their report they detailed the harm their presence in their hosts was causing them. They also elaborated on how the adverse effects of their presence on the health and well-being of their human hosts had in turn led to massive disruption in almost aspect of life on earth.

Chapter 2E
How could King Corona
have anticipated this?!

How could the most august King of Coronaland have anticipated this?! How indeed could the head of the Corona community have foreseen, to have predicted, that their experimental mission to settle with human-kind would have such catastrophic repercussion on humanity?

King Corona was so saddened by the reports of the human suffer-ings, in particular the loss of lives as well as the disruption in life on earth, he considered calling an immediate end to the mission. Easier said than done, as he would soon learn from his top advisers and ex-perts!

Indeed he was told by the experts that, as a result of several factors, a few of which are outlined below, it was virtually impossible for him to call an end to the expedition.

First was the speed at which the seven researcher had managed, within the short time, to replicate themselves within their human hosts. In the horse bats, they usually managed to replicate themselves in small amounts at a time. The abundance of space at their disposal in their human hosts had enabled them within a short time to replicate them-selves in the hundreds of thousands.

The lifestyle of humans, which involves moving quickly from place to place with sophisticated means of travel developed by their complex brains, for example the aeroplane, had already resulted in some of the newcomers being taken to far, distant lands and spread in great numbers to other humans. The seven researchers had even lost contact with them. In such a situation, how could King Corona recall them back home?

As over the next few weeks the researchers continued to relay messages of the suffering, death and economic turmoil that had visited the earth following their incursions into their human hosts, King Corona was so distressed, a time came when he refused to take in meals and fluids. He went on a hunger strike.

After staying away from foods and fluids for a week, he became so emaciated, his subjects feared for his life. In the end, his dear wife, the queen, managed to persuade him to resume eating and drinking again.

Still the thought of the misery caused by his subjects to humanity would not leave him in peace. Over the next several days he continued to tell his subjects: "We should have stayed with our old friends the horse bats and not ventured into the human community. I can only hope and pray humanity will take all the necessary steps and measures to curb the spread of my subjects around the globe."

But will humanity act and behave the way King Corona would have wished? Only time will tell.

Chapter 2F

When speed is of the essence

So Corona had made a successful incursion into humanity. Indeed, within a matter of about three months they had managed to spread to every corner of the globe.

In this chapter an attempt will be made to briefly map out the course of the journeys of the expeditioners from Coronaland around the globe.

Since much of the directions of their travels are already in the public domain, only a brief sketch will be provided here so as to avoid repetition.

Asia

As already noted, the intruders made their first landing in Wuhan, in the Hubei province of China. From there they began to spread to the rest of the country.

Within a matter of days the expeditioners were carried by some of their human host beyond the borders of China to neighbouring countries such as Thailand, South Korea and Japan

Their presence in Japanese territory gained particular international attention by virtue of the involvement of the cruise ship Diamond Princess. The ship had left the port city Yokohama, near Tokyo, on 20 January, for a two-week dream cruise to China, Vietnam, Taiwan and back to Japan. Towards the end of the cruise, an 80-year-old guest who disembarked in Hong Kong on 25 January showed signs of symptoms, which led them to think that it could be due to the presence of the newcomers from Coronaland. The suspicion was confirmed through a test on 1 February.

The *Diamond Princess*, carrying 2,666 guests eventually returned to its starting point, Yokohama, on 3 February. Eventually, the cruise ship became one of the hotspots for the spread of the newcomers. In the end, a total of 704 passenger and crew became infected. Six of the affected, unfortunately, succumbed to the adverse effects caused to their body by the Corona expeditioners.

On 30 January, India confirmed its first case involving the new expeditioners from Coronaland. India, the second most populous country on the planet, was caught in a huge dilemma. The nightmare scenario of the virus racing through such a populous country, leading to the possible deaths of thousands if not millions, was certainly playing on the minds of the leaders, when on 24 March their PM ordered all 1.3 billion people in the country to stay inside their homes for three weeks, giving them only four hours' prior notice! A lockdown of 1.3 billion citizens, with practically no warning, would not be without repercussions! "They should have given us at least 10 days' notice", one frustrated citizen complained in exasperation.

With no work in the cities, hundreds of thousands of the poor, who had migrated from the countryside in search of food, decided to return home rather than stay in the cities and face possible starvation.

"Hunger will kill us before Coronavirus," one of them lamented.

There followed a haphazard and disorganised mass migration from the city into the countryside. Indeed, in the end, several lost their lives not from Corona, but rather through starvation, accidents and, in some cases, suicide.

On 19 February, Iran reported the first confrontation of any of her citizens with the new expeditioners to the human community. This happened in their holy city of Qum. In the end, that country was to bear a heavy burden from the effects of the newcomers from Coronaland – both in the form of lost human lives and disruption to their economic activity.

Europe

The first three cases detected in Europe were reported in France on 24 January 2020, with the onset of symptoms on 17, 19 and 23 January.

By March, Europe had become the epicentre of the problem. Italy in particular, was severely affected. Experts are not agreed on the reason; many however point to its aging population as having been a contributory factor.

Spain, Italy's neighbour to the west, would also end up paying a heavy price in the form of human suffering and deaths caused by the uninvited guests from Coronaland.

Germany initially struggled to cope with the arrival of the impudent microbes on her shores. After the initial shock, however, it managed to put systems in place to fairly well mitigate the effect of the uninvited guests on her territory.

The UK was literally overwhelmed by the invisible newcomers, mainly due to the fact it initially downplayed the havoc the presence of the nasty microscopic expeditioners could cause to their human hosts. Thus, at the time the newcomers made a landing on their shores, they were woefully unprepared.

In the end their PM, who by his words and actions conveyed the impression that the effect of the newcomers on the human body was nothing worse than that of their distant cousins the flu virus, was dealt such a devasting blow he just managed to escaped death by a hair's breadth!

Australia and Oceania

On 25 January 2020, the first case of Coronavirus in Australia was confirmed – a man from Wuhan who travelled from Guangzhou to Melbourne on 19 January. A further three cases were confirmed in Sydney – they all involved individuals who had arrived from China.

New Zealand for her part first confirmed the arrival of the intruders from Coronaland on 28 February 2020.

North America

In the US, the first known case involving the newcomers from Coronaland was confirmed in the Pacific Northwest state of Washington on 20 January. It involved an individual who had returned from Wuhan five days before. In the end, that country was to be heavily hit by the pandemic. Indeed, as the time of going to press at the end of July 2020, the country remains the global epicentre of the pandemic.

Canada for its part confirmed the arrival of the visitors from the Corona country on their shores on 27 January 2020. It involved a person who had returned to Toronto from Wuhan.

Africa

For a while, it appeared as if Africa would be spared the trouble of dealing with the intruders from Coronaland. Well, the "peaceful" state of affairs would not prevail for long.

On 14 February 2020, the first case involving the expeditioners from the Coronavirus kingdom was confirmed on the African continent, namely in Egypt. In the next few days, further cases would be reported in other parts of the continent such as Nigeria, South Africa, Ghana etc. In due time each of the continent's 54 countries was affected.

Does the fact that the body of an average African is permanently and daily exposed to bacteria and virus of all types and kinds – cholera, malaria, salmonella, E-coli, pneumococcus, Ebola, you name it – help them deal better with the new invaders from Coronaland compared with their peers living elsewhere in the globe?

The composer of this report can only sing a song about the matter – especially if he sits down to consider the type of water he used to drink as he was growing up in his small village and all the other germs, parasites and virus he was exposed to!

The bodies of residents who manage to survive the incessant attacks from the microscopic world could aptly be referred to as immune fortresses, bunkers, fortifications etc. capable of warding off attacks from invading agents, however strong, virulent and aggressive they may be!

South America

I will cite the experience of three countries from Latin America to map out the path of the newcomers from Coronaland on that continent.

Brazil: The first case pointing to the newcomers from Coronaland on the South American continent was reported on 26 February from Sao Paulo in Brazil. Eventually the country would become one of the global hotspots of the disease.

Mexico on her part confirmed the presence of the intruders from Coronaland in the country on 28 February. It involved two individuals who had returned to the country from Italy.

Argentina confirmed the first case pointing to the arrival of the expeditioners on her shores on 3 March 2020.

Antarctica

As at the time of compiling this report in the last week of July 2020, none of the expeditioners from Coronaland has been spotted on the Antarctic.

Part three
Time for soul-searching

Introductory note

Did King Corona, at the time of dispatching his expeditioners on their mission – ever reckon with such rapid spread of his explorers to virtually every corner of the globe within such a short time?

Could the monarch of Coronaland, in his wildest dreams, have reckoned with the meteoric, lightning speed at which his explorers would spread to every nook, corner and cranny of the earth?

Yet, that exactly turned out to be the case! Within a relatively short time after their first landing in Wuhan, the newcomers had spread to every corner of the globe. Soon, almost everything on planet earth – cabinet meetings of nations, boardroom meetings of multinational organisations, developments on the stock exchange, the course of mega events the likes of the Olympic games etc. – came to revolve only around the new arrivals from Coronaland.

So what went wrong? What could humanity have done better to prevent the rapid spread of the expeditioners from Coronaland around the world?

Before this freelance reporter of the events proceeds to analyse the matter, he wishes to pass a short comment.

In compiling the report, he laid claim to the artistic freedom everyone living in a free society is entitled to. In the process, he sought to be as objective as can be expected of a layman turned freelance reporter.

He also wants to make it clear to the reader that he does not consider himself an expert in the areas of virology, pandemics, public health etc. So whoever is looking for a more in-depth analysis of the issues – for academic dissertation perhaps – should better contact the relevant sources.

So here we go with the factors that, in the view of the compiler of this report, accounted for the swift spread of the expeditioners from

Coronaland around the globe.

The factors are in the main human-related and can be broadly divided into two: (1) direct and (2) indirect human factors. The direct human factors on their part can further be subdivided into two: (a) those resulting from the actions and inactions of authorities or the powers that be; and (b) those resulting from the actions, inactions, behaviour etc of the general public.

Chapter 3A
The powers that be
giving Corona a free ride

Local authorities at Wuhan suppressing the news of the outbreak

Although as the time of compiling this report in July 2020, Coronavirus is a global issue, at the very beginning it affected a so-called ground zero in a particular location in the city of Wuhan. The team from Coronaland settled in the bodies of a few individuals to start with. Theoretically, the spread could have been curtailed if the eyes of humanity had been able to spot them! Of course, everyone is aware that is not the case – the newcomers were too minute to be detected human eyes!

That fact, undeniably, gave the invaders an advantage over humanity. After a few days – a week perhaps? – their effect on their human host began to be felt. At that stage, individuals such as Dr Li Wenliang began to spread the news. The local authorities in Wuhan, for whatever reasons, sought to downplay the seriousness of the matter, allowing time for the new arrivals to be carried to other parts of the country.

Since Wuhan had become an important economic centre of the world, it is not inconceivable that business people from other parts of the globe who were there on business trips carried the microbes to other parts of the world, even before the alarm bells were officially sounded!

Ill-judged decision to evacuate from China

In an ideal world, a ring fence should have been drawn around the whole of China as soon as it became apparent that the newcomers were provoking aggressive responses in the bodies of humans, to the extent that led to the demise of the victims.

The newcomers were microscopic, unseen by the naked eye. Those harbouring them did not always react to their presence. Even those who reacted to their presence did not do so immediately. In such a situation, the general rule should have been, "Everyone stay where you are!"

Indeed ,whether one was citizen of country A, the most influential and wealthy nation on earth, whether one was from the least influential country Z, the rule should have applied to everyone – to the ordinary tourist who happened to be in China at that time as well as high representatives of their various countries. No one – whether ambassadors of the most might country or the least important – should have been permitted to leave the epicentres.

Whether they wanted to hear it or not, the message that should have gone out would have been the following:

"Fellow citizens, whether by fate or by chance you happen to be where you are. You have to endure everything just the way members of the human race over there are enduring it. So for the next several weeks, you have to be where you are until the storm settles. It could be weeks, it could be months, but that is it. Be strong. In the same manner that our Chinese friends are forced to undergo hard times, unfortunately you also have to prepare yourselves for uncertain times."

Well politicians and leaders are not epidemiologists; they unfortunately have the tendency to act to favour their voters: "No, no! we cannot leave our citizens in harm's way, we got to get them out of China as soon as we can!" Thus various countries took steps to quickly organise charter flights to haul their citizens from the "danger zone" back to "safety" – so to Europe, Australia, North America and elsewhere they were repatriated.

The newcomers from Coronaland – hundreds if not thousands of them were delighted at the golden opportunity offered them to spread to other parts of the globe! So they concealed themselves in the bodies of their various hosts, who at that time where not feeling any symptoms, and travelled with them to their various home countries in the Americas, Europe, Oceania etc.

World leaders going their respective ways instead of working together

The moment it became known that the virus had spread to practically every part of the globe, it should have dawned on those at the helm of world affairs that we were dealing with a global problem and not a national one.

In such a situation, world leaders should have come together and developed a single global strategy to deal with the nasty invaders – intruders who had invaded our homes without our consent – a knock-out blow!

But no! Instead of working as a team, countries went their own way. Not only did they take decisions affecting their respective countries without regard to others, they also began to compete over for access to items, devices, gadgets (hand sanitizers, face masks, ventilators etc.) required in the fight against the condition.

Even a political block such as the EU, which one would have expected would take a common stance, did not do so – at least in the initial stages.

The uncoordinated response of humanity resulted in a situation where 195 different countries of planet earth ended up using 195 different tactics to fight one common challenge facing them!

The expeditioners from Coronaland, no doubt, were delighted at the uncoordinated, haphazard, disorganised and, to some degree, unbefitting responses of humanity towards their incursion into their realm.

Strange and bizarre behaviour of some political leaders

Even as the seriousness of the pandemic became evident due to the deadly course it had taken in the countries like China, Iran, Italy and Spain, some world leaders were downplaying the problem with comments like: "It is just like seasonal flu; it will go away quickly."

Some of the leaders seemed also to have the tendency to show off. They took to the platform to show off instead of dealing with the problem. It came to the point that some leaders even seemed to be playing the role of doctors, prescribing treatment to the rest of the world – in some cases against medical advice.

Conflicting, contradictory, imprecise etc. instructions/signals from some in authority

Some of the world leaders and those in authority did not serve as good examples to emulate by disregarding the rules set by themselves.

In the UK, the chief adviser to the PM breached the government's lockdown rules by travelling 264 miles from his home in London in the south to Durham in the north, despite displaying symptoms of the disease.

Following the public outcry, it was widely expected the PM would dismiss him. But no; the PM himself came out in public to defend the indefensible, flouting of the rules by his own adviser!

In my native Ghana a deputy minister breached Covid-19 protocols, when after testing positive to the virus, he visited a registration centre in his constituency where the compilation of voters' register was taking place, before the period of self-isolation was complete. He was subsequently forced to resign by the president.

Even when it was generally held that facial coverings in public places could help stem the spread of the virus, some leaders were not only flouting the laws themselves, but were encouraging the general population to do exactly the same.

Political interference in therapy as well as scientific research

Instead of giving the scientists the needed space and peace of mind to go about their research activities, some politicians, by their behaviour, piled undue pressure on them.

As someone put it, it led to a situation when press conferences were held to announce "soon-to be expected" breakthroughs in the search for a vaccine and/or cure even before such research findings had been peer-reviewed (verified by independent experts in the field study).

In due course, the less well known chloroquine, which the writer of these lines had on several occasions in his childhood and adult life in Ghana taken to treat malaria, and its "cousin" hydroxychloroquine became "world stars" as they were touted by some leading world leaders for their *proven* effectiveness against the nasty invaders from Coronaland.

Leaders fighting to uphold their national pride at the expense of the common good

Waving high their personal egos and their national flags, some politicians sought to uphold their national pride, instead of the common good.

The UK, for example, turned down the invitation by the EU to join the block in the acquisition of PPE, initially for the reason that they were no longer members of the EU. It is difficult to quantify the number of individual who became positive or lost their lives due to the initial shortages of PPE in the country.

The US for its part decided initially to withdraw funding for the WHO and eventually decided to leave the organisation entirely.

That leads me to the matter of the WHO and how it has been sidelined by several countries during the pandemic. Side-lining the WHO! Which organisation was best suited to spearhead a global initiative, apart from the WHO? Was it not formed on 7 April 1948, for exactly that purpose, to among other things stimulate and advance work on the prevention and control of epidemics and pandemics?

Apart from already having the required network in place globally, the WHO can also claim to have the leading experts in the matter of infectiology, epidemiology and public health.

Of course no human institution is perfect. For reasons best known to themselves some world leaders began to magnify what they perceived as the short-comings of the organisation and used that as excuse to sideline them.

I have outlined some of the factors from the side of those in authority that facilitated the spread of the nasty intruders from Coronaland in our midst. The list, of course is not exhaustive.

I now move on to consider how the actions, behaviours, attitudes, lifestyles etc. of the general public, the actions of you and I, gave the newcomers a free ride, as it were, to ravage through our midst – to travel unhindered through our countries.

Chapter 3B

How the behaviour of
the general public
facilitated the spread of Corona

In the previous section, I outlined some of the factors stemming from those in authority that facilitated the spread of the nasty intruders from Coronaland in our midst.

I now move on to consider how the actions, behaviours, attitudes, lifestyles etc. of the general public, the actions of you and I, gave the newcomers a free ride, as it were, to ravage through our midst – to travel unhindered through our countries.

The egotistic human trait working for the Corona team

In January 2020 the case of a Chinese lady, who boasted on social media of having managed to cheat the temperature scanner at the airport so she could fly to Paris, went viral on social media.

Her own account leaves little doubt in my mind that she was carrying some of the newcomers in her body. Instead of self-isolating at home, she decided to fly the distance from China to France. It is anyone's guess how many people she infected as a result – from the various travel points in China to the plane carrying her, to the airport in Paris, the passengers she travelled with in France, the individuals she came across on the streets and in the restaurants.

Of course, that lady was not the only human being who concealed her infection so as to carry out some "essential" activity.

The Western way of life facilitating the spread of Corona

Western industrialised societies have experienced freedom and prosperity since the end of World War II. 75 years of peace in the Western world has led to a prosperous economy. A liberal democratic system permitting unrestricted movement and freedom of speech has resulted in a population not used to any form of restriction of liberties of any kind. Blessed with EU and US passports that enabled them to travel to almost every corner of the globe without, in most cases, the need to fill a visa application form, those who have the means travel at least once a year on holidays.

Western industrialized societies – oh, what a blessed and very small proportion of the human race!

Then all of a sudden, with practically no forewarning, the audacious and daredevil microbes from Coronaland arrived at their borders.

How much some of their leaders would have prevented entry to the nasty intruders by means of massive concrete fortifications! But no, the expeditioners from Coronaland are no respecters of frontiers! In addition, they brought with them a massive disruption of ordinary daily lives and the curtailment of civil liberties.

Among the restrictions were those involving travelling on holiday. Whereas individuals living in a place like Tookwae, the birth village of my paternal grandfather in Ghana, who had no idea what a passport was, nor had seen an aeroplane in their entire lives, could avoid holidays for the whole of their lifetimes, for their cousins in Western industrialised countries this was a massive restriction on their daily lives.

Then there was the issue of the forced lockdown, which in actual fact amounted to house arrest! Elsewhere on the globe, imposing a strict lockdown on a population may not amount to very much, but for a Western society used to the enjoyment of personal liberties, the freedom to do whatever they wished, it meant a huge curtailment in liberties – which some vehemently opposed.

Prosperity and freedom has led societies in the Western world to develop various pastimes, hobbies, habits etc. that they pursue in their leisure time. So, whereas their forefathers who lived 200 years ago, as well as their cousins living in the developing world in certain areas of the globe, would not consider going to places like restaurants, pubs, theatres, Disneyland etc. as a necessity, their human peers living in prosperous Western societies have come to regard them as part and parcel of their everyday lives, indispensable to their well-being. To ask them to suddenly, without warning, forego such lifestyles, which others see as luxuries, is a really tough call.

Consequently, for a good while, some of their leaders played delaying tactics, wondering how they could prescribe such a bitter pill that would lead to such an unprecedented curtailing of their civil rights.

Thus initially the lockdown in places like Italy, which was experiencing increasingly high infection rates, was half-heartedly enforced. It was when it became apparent that the presence of the newcomers was leading to severe healthcare problems, the demise of many residents, that it dawned on the government as well as the population that they were dealing with a really severe healthcare scare – which required the curtailing of the liberties they had enjoyed for years.

The special American factor worsening an already dire situation

Whereas the factors outlined above could be said to be common to Western industrialised countries in general, a good proportion of their fellow humans in the USA, Uncle Sam, behaved in a manner that set them apart from their peers in other Western countries.

Indeed, whereas a good majority of their peers in Western Europe who enjoy a standard of life and liberties comparable to their own came, generally, to accept the lockdown restrictions, a large proportion of US citizens not only opposed it, but also openly demonstrated against it – citing the First Amendment of the US Constitution, which guarantees freedoms of press, speech, assembly, religion and petition!

The personal message of the composer of this report to the US demonstrators insisting on their constitutional rights to freedom and liberty was as follows:

"My dear human compatriots, much as I sympathise with you for the untold hardships brought about by the lockdown, this is not the time to go about demonstrating against the curtailment of your rights enshrined in your constitution. If there is anyone

71

to be angry with, it is the Coronavirus family. It is indeed those nasty microscopic organisms from Coronaland, that have infringed upon our human rights, that have unilaterally decided to invade humanity, hijacking at will the bodies of humans that come their way to perform their physiological functions. Instead of protesting against the authorities, just pick up your arms and confront the invaders in battle. Deal the invaders a deadly blow and set humankind free from this horrible plague!"

Though politics has come into play in several parts of the globe in considering the best way to tackle the problems rising from the Coronavirus incursion into humanity, the situation seems to have been blown out of all proportion in the country of Uncle Sam.

I may be wrong in my assessment, but it appears to me, as an outside observer, that their Republican president in particular and the other Republican governors, seem to want to oppose any measures proposed by their compatriots, the Democrats.

Indeed, whereas most of the Democratic-led states lean towards adopting measures the majority of countries in the world have embarked upon/adopted, their Republican counterparts are more inclined towards a more "liberal" approach, giving the individual the liberty to do as they think fit.

A typical example is the issue of wearing a face mask or facial covering. For a while there has been a tussle going on between those who favour it, made up in the main of politicians from the Democratic camp, and their Republican counterparts who oppose it.

A Kenyan proverb has it that "when elephants fight, it is the grass that suffers". That can aptly be said of the situation in the US concerning the rapid spread of the Corona expeditioners in that country. Indeed, whereas the two political camps wrestle it out as to how best to tackle the problem, the populace are bearing the brunt of the pandemic in the form of lost lives, personal suffering, disruption to formal daily life etc.

It is heart-breaking, really pathetic, to watch the world's so-called remaining superpower, the country that is armed to the teeth with a good proportion of the most sophisticated weapons at the disposal of humanity, torn apart, completely humiliated by just mere microbes from Coronaland!

Miscellaneous factors

Several other human factors bordering on economics, opportunism, complacency etc. favoured the spread of the newcomers around the world.

Football matches and other sporting activities that should have been cancelled or played behind closed doors, were played in full capacity stadia in several places in Europe just at the time when infection was ravaging through the continent.

As touched upon earlier, political pressure led to the evacuation of citizens from affected countries back to their homelands. In some cases some of the evacuees who had tested negative before departing China tested positive on their arrival or shortly thereafter, meaning they could have spread the virus to their co-travellers or those they came in contact with on their arrival.

In the UK, mass events, such as the Cheltenham horse racing meeting, were also allowed to go ahead. That event took place between 10 and 13 March, and was attended by a quarter of a million people from various countries, at about the time when the infection was peaking in several European countries. Experts have spoken about the fact of the event accelerating the spread of the newcomers from Coronaland in the UK and beyond.

Chapter 3C
Indirect human factors
facilitating the spread of Corona

The indirect human factors stem in the main from elements, structures, systems etc. already in place on planet earth prior to the arrival of the expeditioners from Coronaland and which turned out to facilitate their spread around the globe.

An interconnected world serving the cause of the Corona expeditioners

Over the years the world has become increasingly interconnected. Whereas a few decades ago, hardly any travel occurred between, for example, China and the rest of the world, the situation is now different in a world that is now aptly referred to by many as a "global village".

At the time of the arrival of the uninvited guests, international trade was booming. China, where the virus first appeared, had become one of the largest centres of international trade. Wuhan, the city where the newcomers from Coronaland made their landing, had become a trading hub between China and the rest of the world.

Social media's helping hand for Corona

Though it is difficult to establish how much effect it had on the course of the disease and how much it affected compliance with the lockdown rules of various countries, the spread of fake news, disinformation and conspiracy theories in regard to the origin of the disease and its negative impact cannot be ignored.

The internet, whilst being overwhelmingly a blessing to the world, served as a welcome tool for those bent on spreading false news, misinformation, conspiracy theories etc.

It is not clear the extent to which the fake news, disinformation, conspiracy theories and other bizarre allegations and wild rumours circulating online and by means of other agents of mass communication facilitated the travel of the expeditioners from Coronaland through the world. It is not inconceivable, though, that those who believed them would be among those who were likely not to adhere to the recommended preventive measures and, in so doing, help to spread the disease.

Adverse effects of "warehousing" the elderly

Even if the practice of keeping the old in residential home did not directly contribute to the spread of the newcomers among the human population, it contributed to the high death toll. The congregation of the elderly and vulnerable in an enclosed space no doubt facilitated the spread of the virus amongst the residents, whose frail body systems turned out to be incapable of coping with the sudden and unexpected extra burden imposed on their health by the uninvited visitors from Coronaland.

Poverty and deprivation

In many places in the developing world, residents live in crowded, dilapidated settlements, which in some cases can be aptly described as "unfit for human habitation". Such individuals live from hand to mouth. As someone put it, "if a bird does not fly, it does not eat". Indeed with hardly any social welfare system in place to cater for them in case of ill health, such individuals are virtually lost.

How does anyone expect such groups of individuals to maintain social distancing and abide by the lockdown protocols put in place in several places at the height of the pandemic, without making provisions for the replacement of the income they will have to forgo?

I watched a TV report on how the poor and deprived of India were coping with the Coronavirus lockdown. As one of those stricken by poverty explained: "Many of us share the same toilet, we are crammed in the same rooms, how do we maintain social distancing under such conditions?"

Among the poor, many were forced outside to leave home in search for their daily bread and in the process either became infected or passed on the infection to others.

The above, and several other factors that have not been touched upon for the sake of space and time, have facilitated the spread of the Corona expeditors, who, as we remember, arrived in the human community as group of seven expeditioners!

Part four
Corona is here to stay

Chapter 4A
The gist of a 100-page report

As had been planned at beginning of their incursions to earth, at the end of the sixth month of their stay with humanity, the expeditioners sent with humanity, the expediters sent their final report to their king. The crux of the 100-page report was that they were here to stay. In humans they feel comfortable; they have much more space to go about their activities.

They only wish that humanity would have a way to accommodate them, that they were able better to tolerate them – just as in the case of the horse bats. They did not come with the intention to destroy them, cause their deaths. Neither is it in their interests to disrupt the economic livelihood of their human hosts.

Part of the population would still stay with the horse bats and other non-human creatures, whilst the others would remain with mankind. It was part of their long-term survival strategy to spread their risks in an unsecure and unpredictable world. It was a precautionary measure, to ensure their survival. Should something happen to cause the extinction of one of their host, they could still fall on the other to maintain their existence on earth..

The human population for their part had come to accept the fact that, however unpleasant it might sound to their ears, they may have to reckon with the presence of the intruders in their community for the foreseeable future.

Indeed as at the time of going to press at the end of July 2020, officially, it has infected 16.5 million of the world's population and led to the deaths of over 650,000 people. It is generally held that the actual number of the infected could be double the official figure.

Since the expeditioners from Coronaland are already established on earth, the question worthy of asking as at the time of compiling this report at the end of July 2020 is – what next for humanity? What is the way forward for the global human community?

Humanity, without doubt is confronted with the most challenging healthcare as well as socio-economic crisis since the end of World War II.

All the experts agree that the only way life on earth can return to normalcy, a state of affairs comparable to what it was prior to the emergence of Coronavirus, is to develop an effective vaccine and/or cure.

As of 31 July 2020, though there has been some encouraging news concerning the search for a vaccine, the experts agree that it might take several months before such a vaccine is licensed. And even should a vaccine become available, it would without doubt take a while before it becomes available to each of the approximately 7.8 billion inhabitants of earth.

It can thus be said that in the short and medium term, humanity has had to find a way of dealing with the havoc brought about by the expeditioners from Coronaland.

Chapter 4B
The humble contributions
of a concerned citizen

I, the composer of this report, wish once again to lay claim to my artistic freedom to make my humble contribution as to how humanity could defeat this uninvited guests causing deaths and untold suffering to humanity. I will in this connection resort to some of the experience I gained learning an apprenticeship in the field of medical sciences.

Before I present my input, I want to pass a short comment. There is a saying that no one can claim monopoly on wisdom. So I want to make it known that I am not claiming expertise in the matter. If after reading through my lines you find my ideas silly, nothing for the intelligent mind, you can please discard everything. You may use your artistic freedom to write the most scathing of reviews about it. I am begging though that we allow everything to play out on the level of civility, that we behave politely to each other. After all, the problem at stake is not the making of you and I. Rather it is the fault of these insolent microbes that have taken it upon themselves to interfere in our way of live in such abhorrent, detestable manner. So here we go.

I want to consider the matter from the short-, medium- and long-term perspectives.

Short and medium term

It will involve a nine-month period from the beginning of September 2020 until the end of May 2021.

Before I go into the details of my proposals, I want to pass a short comment. As I indicated above, all the experts agree that the best way out of the present situation is the development of a vaccine, which, even if it does not provide 100% protection, would be able to provide a reasonably good protection to help the body cope with an infection in a manner that would avert the development of severe disease symptoms warranting hospital treatment.

From what I am hearing and reading from the experts, it appears unlikely that such a vaccine will be available in the course of 2020 – which makes it quite likely that a second wave of infection could, in the coming autumn and winter months, visit Europe and several places in the northern hemisphere where the infection rate seems to have receded considerably.

As someone put it, as we hope for the best, we need to prepare for the worst. So how do we prepare for the immediate future, with the possibility of a second infection wave in mind?

I would want to propose a radical approach to the problem. Before I provide further details on the matter, I want to digress a bit to use an example from medical practice to illustrate my point.

When a doctor is consulted about a medical condition, the learned fellow usually takes the history of the patient and subsequently carries out a clinical examination and performs various test to develop a therapy and treatment plan. There are several forms of therapy. It is not the remit of this book to go into details – I will only provide an overview. Therapy could be conservative, which involves resorting to non-surgical means such as medication, injections, physiotherapy, etc., as well as surgery. Surgery for its part can be simple – which is usually restricted to the affected organ, or radical, which could be extended to other neighbouring organs/structures.

There are instances when surgery is carried out not with the aim of curing the patient, but rather in the context of providing palliative relief. For example, when a tumour that is deemed incurable happens to be compressing an important organ leading to the impairment in the function of the affected organ, surgery could be conducted, not with the goal of cure, but of bringing about an improvement in the quality of life of the patient.

Indeed, to help humanity defeat this nasty virus for good, I would adopt a very radical approach, which in my view is the best possible way to overcome the virus and reduce to the barest minimum the risk of the virus keeping on recurring/emerging at intervals – short or long– to cause us problems.

Below then is my plan:

The plan would involve taking responsibility in the management of the pandemic away from politicians and placing it into the hands of an international task force of highly regarded healthcare professionals working under the auspices of the WHO.

The WHO will play a key role in the plan I am proposing.

Indeed, despite any shortfalls they are accused of – real, exaggerated, imagined etc. – the organisation is the only one I know that has the needed network in place over the globe to handle the matter.

For goodness sake, why should the world sideline the very organisation we created to deal with a pandemic of this type? The politicians who are making a career criticising them are creating the impression they themselves are without fault. He who is without fault please throw the first stone at the WHO!

The task force would have the last say in every decision directly connected with the management of the pandemic globally. They would be free from any political intervention, gimmicks, adventurism, showmanship, and what have you.

Under the proposed plan, every country would appoint at least one top healthcare expert – chosen for their competency and not out of political considerations, affiliations, loyalty etc. – to serve on the task force.

Though I do not want to interfere in the internal affairs of other countries, I would humbly suggest that in the case of the United States, Dr Fauci should head any team of experts chosen to represent that country on the proposed task force.

I listened to an interview he gave on BBC Radio 4 at the beginning of July on how to manage pandemics in general and the current one in particular. After listening to his input, my spontaneous reaction was: "Whoa! These are the kinds of experts, the types of healthcare gurus – individual, who have been dealing with such type of outbreaks for the greater part of their professional life, individuals to whom fighting such infections can be regarded as their 'daily bread' – who should be entrusted with responsibility for the management of this awful pandemic."

The healthcare experts will have the final say in measures needed to fight the pandemic from the medical/healthcare perspective.

If, for example, they decide that based on the prevailing infection figures the whole of the United States or Brazil or Nigeria should be sent to lock down, that is exactly what should happen.

The international taskforce will manage the healthcare aspect, based on the best evidence, and leave the politicians the responsibility of sorting out the economic repercussions of the decision of the healthcare experts, and also explaining to the populace why they have had to take decisions, however harsh, based on the recommendations of the healthcare experts.

Such an arrangement would even work to the advantage of the politicians, since they could rightly shift responsibility to the healthcare experts, who, I dare conjecture, would not be bothered by public pressure since they do not depend on them for their votes – and since they would be working with a clear conscience based on the latest scientific evidence, they would not have cause to worry.

In this regard, I would strongly recommend the complete adoption of the United Nations Development Programme report published on their website, www.undp.org on 23 June 2020 calling for the introduction of a temporary basic income (TBI) to provide "a minimum guaranteed income above the poverty line, for vulnerable people in 132 developing countries", to quote directly from the UNDP report. Such income will allow 2.7 billion people who come under that category to stay at home.

I will suggest that the TBI provision is put in place in time to coincide with the start of work of the Global Coronavirus Eradication Taskforce (GCET) on 1 September. The emergency assistance should be paid out for a period of nine months, subject to extension.

I also propose that during the nine-month period no report on the ongoing research into a vaccine and cure for Covid-19 is put into the public domain until such time that it has undergone a peer review of independent experts.

That indeed is what has been the common practice so far. How many types of research into various health conditions – cancer, dementia, Alzheimer etc. –are going on behind the scenes, without public knowledge? Why should the research into Covid-19 be treated differently? Indeed why should the public be informed about any minute insight gained at every stage of the research into vaccine and a cure? Scientist and experts in the area could be kept in the loop, not though the general public.

Indeed, much as I do accept the huge public interest in the development of a vaccine and/or cure for the healthcare problems arising from the incursions of the loathsome, dreadful microbes from Coronaland, in my opinion, the research process should not be different from any other scientific research. In my opinion, it is better to wait till the most decisive stage – the stage where a vaccine or drug has cleared all the research hurdles and is about to be licensed for use, before the enchanting news of a breakthrough in the "fight" against Coronavirus is splashed across the airwaves.

That will prevent a situation where hopes would be raised in the public regarding the imminent arrival of a vaccine or cure, only for it to be dashed in no time.

Though I cannot provide any figures to back my case, I do think such false hopes can also lead some in the general public to disregard preventive measures. Reading from a mass circulation newspaper about a vaccine possibly becoming available in a few months' time may lead some to think we have got on top of the problem, and lead them to disregard the precautionary measure expected from them to help contain the virus.

My several years' experience as a family doctor has led me to appreciate how much influence media reports are taken seriously, without a pinch of salt, by a section of the general public. Lay people as they are in the matters of medical science, some in the general public tend indeed to believe media reports on alleged new insights into the cure of diseases.

I have lost count of the number of times that I have been confronted with the following: "Doc, I read this and that in the newspapers, heard this and that on radio, saw this and that on TV concerning the effective cure to this and that ailment through this and that medication. Can you please prescribe it for me?!"

My proposal may not gain majority support. Still in my view there is no other way we could better beat this nasty Coronavirus but through a concerted action by an international team of experts and scientists.

What is desirable: a radical, concerted effort, which may cause pain and discomfort in the short term, but eventually helps us to subdue the virus or an inconsistent, vacillating, haphazard, roller-coaster approach, which keeps us, as it were, going around in circles all the time – today we ease lockdowns, flood to the beach, travel on holidays only to be sent back to lockdown due to a surge in infections.

Without the invention of an effective vaccine to break the cycle, we might have to brace ourselves for that type of situation for the next serval years. We could indeed go around in circles for God knows how long!

Even if the powers that be do not go with the radical approach I am proposing, in the short and medium term –indeed, until we find an effective vaccine and/or cure – every one of the 195 or so world leaders would have to come to terms with the fact that Covid-19 is a global problem that needs a co-ordinated global approach. Such international co-operation is indeed essential, vital, so long as we have not found a vaccine and/or a cure for the condition.

In this connection, my plea to world leaders is that we put all squabbles aside and channel our efforts through the WHO. A concerted effort of the WHO and expert infectiologists and epidemiologist such as Dr Fauci from member countries presents the world the best chance of getting a grip on the ravaging pandemic.

It is also imperative that national leaders listen to any advice that the WHO, working in conjunction with the experts from their respective countries, have for their individual countries.

With all due respects to our political leaders, the bottom line is that this pandemic is a healthcare issue and not a political one. Some of our leaders may be competent political scientists, economists, legal experts, journalists, etc. You deserve unreserved admiration for the knowledge you acquired through hard work at university and other institutions of high learning. The bottom line, however, is that Covid-19 is a medical issue, falling under the sphere of doctors, nurses, public health experts etc.

I want to reiterate – please, honourable leaders of our various countries, on behalf of the world community, I am pleading to you to keep your egos and personal political ambitions in check and listen to the expert advice, give the experts the free hand they need to carry out their professional duties. Indeed, in the absence of an effective vaccine and/or a cure, there is no other way I can envisage a way out of our present situation other than keeping to the advice of the experts in the matter.

Many of us are looking forward to the Olympic games, rescheduled for summer 2021 as well as the football world cup in 2022. Well, without dealing with the matter collectively, we might as well bury our dreams, for how could we organise such events if every country has not managed to bring their infection rates down to acceptable numbers – if not completely eradicate them

Even if, thank goodness, we get an effective vaccine, there is no guarantee it could offer 100% protection or, even if it does initially, there is no guarantee the virus would not undergo mutation that would render what was considered an effective vaccine unreliable or ineffective after a short while and bring us back to square one and require a search for an entirely new vaccine or a modified version of the old one.

The aggressive invaders from Coronaland have indeed brought about a situation that requires everyone, whether we like it or not, to work together.

"Publish or perish" is an aphorism or saying that alludes to the pressure on researchers to publish academic work in order to advance in an academic career. Successful publications bring attention to scholars and their sponsoring institutions, which can facilitate continued funding and with it their careers. Concerning humanity's dealing with the Corona expeditioners, I would beg to modify the above aphorism as follows: "cooperate or perish".

It would definitely be overblown and hype to state that the invaders from Corona will be in a position to bring about a complete annihilation of the human race. Nevertheless, unless humankind co-operates, co-ordinates our efforts towards containing the problem, the impudent invaders could lead us around by the nose for a considerable while!

Indeed it is illusionary for any country to think they could, in the long term, solve the problem on their own. The cases of some countries I do not want to mention by name which publicly celebrated their presumed victory over the virus, only to witness a resurgence only a few weeks later, underscores my point.

Long term

The long-term approach could be considered from two viewpoints – the gloomy, pessimistic perspective and the hopeful, optimistic point of view.

The awful prospect of life in a world without an antidote for Covid-19

I want, firstly, to consider the bleakest prospect of humanity being incapable of developing a vaccine and/or finding a cure for the condition. I have heard highly placed experts in the area of virology raising those concerns. Their concerns are based on the fact that almost 40 years on, humanity is yet to find a vaccine for the human immunodeficiency virus (HIV), which causes the acquired immunodeficiency syndrome (AIDS).

Some are also pointing to the fact the Coronavirus that causes Covid-19 is not the only type of Coronavirus that has "attacked" humanity in recent times. They point in this connection to types of Coronavirus that caused the severe acute respiratory syndrome (SARS) outbreak in 2002. As at now there are no licensed vaccines for that condition.

There is much discussion within the expert community on the matter.

Concerning HIV, the experts are saying a vaccine has not been developed due mainly to the fact that it attacks the host immune system, making it difficult to design an effective vaccine. Besides that, it also mutates rapidly, diversifying within a person over the course of their infection.

Concerning the Coronavirus associated with the SARS outbreak, the experts point to the fact that following its emergence in 2002, SARS, the disease they caused, was quickly contained. While several SARS vaccine candidates were developed, funding dried up preventing the research to be carried to the final conclusion.

The situation is different in the case of Covid-19. I dare say that apart from those who by virtue of age are too young to understand their environment or too advanced in age to be in control of their cognitive functions, or those who due to various medical conditions that have been impaired in speech and mental functions as to know what is going on around them, the word Coronavirus, Covid-19, is in the minds and mouth of each of the 7.8 billion earth residents.

Covid-19, the disease associated with the novella Coronavirus, has indeed brought indescribable suffering and massive disruption to life on earth. That fact has helped ignite our determination to defeat it.

One might imagine the situation where we have let well over a hundred hungry cats loose in pursuance of a single impudent mouse, which has been behaving insolently, ravaging our home with impunity, bringing in the process much devastation to our home and property. It might well be considered magical, unimaginably paranormal, if it does indeed manage to outwit its pursuers and stay alive!

The analogy might well be transposed to humanity's ongoing search for an antidote against the problems brought about by the new-comers from Coronaland. Indeed as I write, researchers worldwide are working around the clock to find a vaccine against the SARS-CoV-2, the virus causing the pandemic. There are said to be over 100 such re-searches going on, of which 40 are thought to be in various advanced stages of development. The huge effort being undertaken globally in the search for a remedy for Covid-19 has made me think we could in-deed get a vaccine and/or cure in the course of 2021.

If, despite such massive efforts on our part to find a remedy against Covid-19, success fails to crown our efforts, then humanity could find itself in real trouble. It is such a depressing outlook – I just do not want to ponder it!

What, in such a situation, will be the future of such major events as the Olympic Games, world athletics meetings, the football World Cup etc.

What will become of world aviation and travel?

How will the composer of these lines, sat in front of my laptop in a small town in the English Midlands, in her Majesty's Kingdom of

Great Britain and Northern Ireland, ever hope of going back home to visit the small village of my birth, Mpintimpi in Ghana, should the airports remain closed due to Corona? Venture by way of the sea route, perhaps? Well, I could give it a try. But what would happen if the nasty invaders from Coronaland give us chase, and grasped all on board by the necks, threatening to suffocate us on the high sea!

May Almighty God, please preserve humankind from such an horrific scenario –a situation whereby we are forced to live indefinitely with the invaders from Coronaland with no vaccine or cure at our disposal.

The joyful prospect of defeating Covid-19

An effective vaccine, supported by medication that could be used to treat those who contract the disease despite an inoculation or those who miss or even refuse the vaccination is what is the world is hoping for, a prospect that could help return life on earth to how it used to be prior to the emergence of the newcomers from Coronaland.

Talking of those who may reject the vaccination: even as we look optimistically into the future, hoping for the development of an effective vaccine for Covid-19, we should not lose sight of a small but fervent group of anti-vaccination activists campaigning against it! Resorting to outlandish arguments and narratives, they are calling for their supporters to reject this or any other type of vaccine. It's not known how many people would actually follow their advice. But their potential for undermining efforts at getting on top of the current pandemic through such unwarranted actions cannot be underestimated.

Chapter 4C
Gearing ourselves for the inevitable

Even if humanity is able to come up with an effective vaccine and/or a cure for Covid-19, and if the efforts of the anti-vaccine campaigners do not negatively impact it, all the experts agree that this is certainly not going to be the last time humanity will face a global pandemic with an agent of a similar or even more potent virulence.

Indeed, at the beginning of July 2020, a report circulated to the effect that another virus with the potential to causing a pandemic of the same if not worse magnitude had been isolated in pigs in China!

Those of us who have seen the wrinkles begin to develop in our faces from ageing may probably not live to witness it. Not so those who are presently in their teens and early twenties. Well, my dear ones, you may well be called upon again to obey lockdown regulations due to another virulent virus pandemic!

Please do not take me to be a prophet of doom! I am only basing my predictions on what the gurus in the matter of virology are reporting.

Humanity is thus best advised to plan for the long haul. What needs to be done?

There is a saying that no one has the monopoly on wisdom. In this vein, I want to make my humble contribution to the debate.

Having grown up in the most humble of conditions, I will, in this connection, bring the perspective of the poor into the debate. Indeed the world tends to forget the poor in such discussions. Let us just sit down to consider the matter. The poor, those who live under the minimum subsistence standards of the UN, make up about a third of the world's population, yet when it comes to matters pertaining to their affairs, hardly anyone thinks about them. Indeed, most of what I have read concerning how to prevent and manage pandemics is written from the point of view of our cousins in the industrialised world – we must do this or that to maintain capital, stabilise our economy.

For that reason in particular, I want to start my contribution on how best to prepare for a future pandemic from the point of view of the poor.

A call for a global "Marshall Plan" against poverty

If the world wants to better position itself to manage or contain future pandemics, we need to embark on appropriate measures towards the eradication of abject poverty from the surface of the earth.

If we want to lessen the chances of a pandemic, especially a respiratory pandemic such as Coronavirus, recurring in the future, we need to take steps to prevent citizens from living in overcrowded dilapidated settlements. Such a situation, in my view, should no longer be regarded as the internal problem of developing countries, but rather a global healthcare issue.

How do we solve the problem? I am calling for a global action plan, a type of Marshall Plan (which was also known as the European Recovery Program, a US program providing aid to help rebuild western Europe following the devastation of World War II).

This global "Marshall Plan" will call for the construction of decent homes for the very poor – so as to enable them to maintain the basic hygiene required to prevent the emergence and subsequent spread of disease.

During the current pandemic, the world requires from the poor that they keep to the protocol on distancing. If that is the case, we need to build them suitable homes to enable them to keep to what is being demanded of them.

We cannot sit in our offices or hotels and prescribe something that is not implementable on the ground.

The rich nations should not consider their contribution to the project/endeavour as a favour they are doing the poor. I see it as a matter of the survival of our human race. It is not polemic.

Of course, if we are going to consider such measures, the world community should find a way of circumventing the corrupt leaders at-the helm of the affairs of the countries where most of the poor of the world reside. We need to prevent a situation where the monies ear-marked by the global Marshall Plan for the construction of homes and other measures aimed at poverty alleviation end up in the pockets of their corrupt leaders.

A call for pandemic hospitals

Countries should establish what I will describe as pandemic hospitals as a way of preparing for future pandemics of a kind similar to the in-fluenza pandemic of 1918 and the Covid-19 pandemic of 2020.

Such hospitals should be particularly equipped to deal with respiratory pandemics that spread quickly. Such centres will not be left idle in "peace" time, those periods when humanity are left in peace by our death-bringing microscopic foes. Instead, such centres would operate as normal hospitals in normal times, only to resume their original function at short notices when required.

The weakness in our preparedness for attacks from the microscopic world was laid bare during the current pandemic. Indeed whereas countries boasted huge stockpiles of arms to fight wars with our perceived human enemy, many struggled to supply mere face masks and gloves for their healthcare staff.

Together we stand, divided we fall

The fact that we live on one and the same planet and that there are myriads of microscopic organism capable of attacking us has, hopefully, dawned on everyone

So what is the best way for humanity to meet the challenges from the microscopic world? Together we stand, divided we fall is an old adage; it is applicable in this situation as well.

It is indeed an illusion for any country to assume they can be an island in this fight with the microscopic word.

There have been pandemics in the past. The difference between today's world and the world of previous pandemics is how very interconnected we have become.

During the last major pandemic of 1968, which was caused by an influenza (H3N2) virus, and led to an estimated one million deaths worldwide, the world was divided into east and west, travel between eastern Europe and the rest of the world was not so developed. Not much in the way of travel took place between Africa and the rest of the world. Communist China permitted hardly any of her citizens to travel around the world.

Today we live in a global village, not only by virtue of the internet. When I attended my father's funeral one of the mourners in attendance was a Chinese lady who happened to reside in a neighbouring town. She decided to accompany her Ghanaian business partner to the event in her desire to familiarize herself with our culture.

Indeed we are today as connected globally as never before. So whether we like it or not we are condemned to work together.

The whole of Europe could get rid of the last Coronavirus from their shores. But so long as it is not eradicated from Africa or the US or China, they dare not toast the final victory.

The best way mankind can deal with pandemics is to assume a common front. In this regard, it is important, as already stressed, that they strengthen the WHO, assign the world organisation a central role not only in the fight against but also the prevention of future pandemics.

Long overdue: a second look at the concept of "defence"

I could be in the minority, but after all the havoc caused by Covid-19, in view of the humiliation inflicted on humankind by this pandemic, I ask whether nations still have to spend huge sums of money piling up arms in preparedness for conflict between themselves?

Instead of nations spending billions on arms shouldn't they instead invest resources in beefing up the world healthcare systems, which have proven woefully inadequate in the current pandemic?

I read the other day that Corona has led to many more deaths in the US than all the wars they have fought since the end of World War II. That alone should call for a rethink and re-appraisal of the strategic defence planning of nations.

Other matters to consider

Since the Coronavirus made a leap from wildlife into the human population there are increasingly loud calls for a ban in the hunting and sale of wildlife.

Still others are calling for a rethink in the practice of mass production of animals such as fowls, pigs, sheep in enclosed spaces for human consumption.

My view as a person who is not an expert in the area is that such proposals, whilst laudable, might well be classified as "easier said than done".

How can I demand from an impoverished resident somewhere on earth who has no other alternative, than to resort to such practice to feed themselves and their family to forego what amounts to their source of existence, unless I make provisions for an alternative means of sustenance?

Well, since it is not my area of expertise, I don't want to delve any deeper into the matter. It brings us really back to the matter of the need for the world community to work together going forward. If indeed the rich countries are ready to dip into their pockets to provide alternative means of sustenance to such individuals, then of course I will readily come on board.

As already indicated, I do not consider myself an authority in the area so I will leave it to those for whom finding solutions to such challenges could be considered their daily bread.

For now, however, I am closing the chapter to retire to bed. I am indeed really exhausted from so much thinking and writing; so, good night dear fellow earth dweller!

Appendix

The ABCs of the novel Coronavirus disease, aka Covid-19

I want to state at the onset that I am not an expert in this matter, so this is not the ultimate authority on the topic. I have however consulted relevant literature. So this can regarded as, of today, 31 July 2020, fairly up-to-date information. So here we go. Let's begin with the basics:

A virus – a mere particle or a living being?

There is no consensus among the experts as to whether a virus is a living being or just a particle. What is beyond contention is that viruses cannot exit on their own – they need a host medium to carry out their activities. There are several types of viruses; they infect not only animals but also plants. Concerning the Coronavirus, there a few types of their kind. In 2003, one type caused the diseases that came to be known as SARS (severe acute respiratory syndrome).

Indeed when residents of Wuhan began to seek medical help for the mysterious respiratory condition afflicting them, doctors initially thought it was another SARS outbreak.

The Coronavirus family derive their name "Corona" by virtue of the fact that they look like "crowns" when viewed under the microscope.

Symptoms of the disease

Covid-19 may not initially cause any symptoms for some people; studies have shown that some affected could carry it for up to two weeks without displaying symptoms.

Some of the common symptoms of the condition are: fever, cough, sore throat, muscle aches and pain, loss of taste and smell. More severe symptoms include the following: shortness of breath/trouble breathing, blue lips or face, persistent pain or pressure in the chest, confusion, excessive drowsiness.

It is generally held that individuals with pre-conditions or underlying medical problems such as heart and circulatory conditions, diabetes, diseases affecting breathing such as asthma, cancer, HIV, obesity (being overweight) are more at risk of experiencing a severe outcome of the infection.

How is the virus spread?

The virus is usually spread directly from an infected person to others by way of droplets in the air following coughing, sneezing or talking.

The viral material hangs out in these droplets and can be breathed into the respiratory tract (your windpipe and lungs), where the virus can then lead to an infection.

It can also be spread by way of the airborne route in the absence of an infected person. In other words the droplets carrying the viruses are capable of flowing about in the air for a while before evaporating or vanishing, long after the infected person has left the scene.

One could also catch the virus after touching a surface or object that has the virus and then touching the mouth, nose, or eyes.

Hoping for a vaccine and/or cure

There is so far no treatment for the disease. Treatment aims at addressing symptoms, such as fever, muscle aches, headaches, shortness of breath etc. Severe cases may require hospitalisation and support such as mechanical ventilation.

Antiviral medications are currently being tested to see if they can address symptoms. Some well-known medication, for example the steroid betamethasone, are said to lead to a more favourable outcomes in hospitalised patients displaying severe disease symptoms.

Vaccine: At the time of going to press at the end of July 2020, there have been clinical trials of a few of the several vaccines in development. Though some have been reported as showing encouraging results, the earliest many experts reckon with the actual licensing of any of them for use is in the course of 2021.

Prevention is better than cure

In the absence of a vaccine and/or a cure, measures aimed at disease prevention are the most effect weapon at the disposal of humanity. These involve adherence to general hygienic measures and other protocols aimed at reducing person-to-person transmission such as:

- frequent hand washing and/or sanitising
- avoiding touching the face, eyes, nose, or mouth with dirty hands
- keeping social distancing rules
- wearing facial covering in public places
- sneezing or coughing in a tissue or in the elbow when in public places
- disposing of any tissues coughed or sneezed into right away.
- routinely disinfecting objects one comes into frequent contact with – phones, computers, and doorknobs etc.

"Physician heal thouself!"

Since there is as yet no vaccine and/or cure for Coronavirus, it may be helpful to learn from how others overcame their infection. With that in mind, I am sharing with the public the measures I embarked upon and adopted when I had a personal encounter with what I have all along referred to in my narration as the expeditioners from Coronaland.

Since a section of humanity tends to be legalistic, I want hereby to declare through this disclaimer that I am not an authority on the matter of Covid-19 treatment and that no one is obliged to emulate my example.

I experienced the first signs of disease on Saturday 28 March. The initial symptoms were fever, sore throat as well as general muscle pain.

In the seven days prior to the begin of my symptoms, I had worked in two different prisons. I worked in one of the prisons exactly a week before the onset of my symptoms and the other on the Monday and Tuesday before.

Did I catch it in one of the two establishments? Since I travelled to work alone in my vehicle and since no one in the family had any symptoms, my guess is that that was likely the case.

At the time I developed the symptoms, community testing for Covid-19 had been abandoned. For the sake of the layman in medicine, I want to pause for a while to explain the two types of tests that can be carried following an infection with an organism such as virus or bacteria.

The first test detects the actual presence of the intruder in the body. The second test is usually carried out a few weeks after exposure to the organism to test for antibodies. The presence of antibodies specific to the agent in question would confirm such exposure. It must be said that some may be exposed to the agent without developing any symptoms. The presence of antibodies at a later date would confirm such an encounter. I do not want to delve into any further details, in order not to confuse the lay person in such matters.

Much as I would have wished to undergo the first test to confirm or exclude infection, I could not do so due to test inaccessibility.

The UK government decided to stop community testing for the virus on 7 March 2020. Though I would have willingly paid for the test myself, they were not generally available outside the state-run National Health Service (NHS).

Although I had Covid-19 at the back of my mind, initially I took it for seasonal flu. Thinking it was flu, I treated it the way I have been treating my flu-like symptoms over the years – treating the symptoms of muscle pain and fever whilst at the same time boosting the body defence system to deal with the infection.

Talking of the body's defence system, the immune system in place in our bodies is constantly fighting against germs and other foreign bodies that manage to enter our body system. Put another way, long before the novel Coronavirus emerged from the blue and captured the world's headlines, our immune system had been fighting all sorts of bacteria, viruses, pollutants etc. Indeed, even without noticing it, our body defence system has been preserving us from harm. Indeed, the body defence system of some of you who are reading these lines might have dealt with a battalion of Coronavirus that attacked you a few days ago, or is even in the process of attacking you right now as you are reading theses line in 2020 without you even noticing them! You better take your gallant soldiers out for a meal in appreciation of their bravery!

Now back to my case. Concerning the control of symptoms of fever, sore throat and bodily aches I initially I resorted to aspirin plus vitamin C soluble tablets as well as multivitamins. I want to provide a short background to that. Prior to settling in the UK, I had spent a little over 20 years in Germany. During that time, I had developed the habit of treating my common flu symptoms that way – which helped in most cases. Since our move to the UK, we travel back to Germany frequently. Whenever we are there, we purchase a stock of such over-the-counter medication.

Thus at the time I developed the symptoms that turned out to be Covid-19 I had enough stock of aspirin plus vitamin C and multivitamin soluble tablets on me to last for several days.

Initially I took two aspirin plus vitamin C soluble tablets three times as well as two multivitamin soluble tablets daily (which amounted to 3 grams of aspirin daily).[1]

I felt so generally unwell I spent much of Saturday and Sunday in bed. There is talk of persistent dry cough being one of the symptoms. In my case though coughing was not pronounced. When I realised during the course of Sunday, that taking aspirin alone was not helping to reduce the temperature, which hovered around 38.6 degrees Celsius, I decided to add paracetamol (known elsewhere as acetaminophen). Though it helped reduce the temperature, it rarely got below 38 degrees Celsius.

My agency had booked me to work the following Monday through to Wednesday. Still thinking it could be common flu (sometimes flu can also be quite stubborn and will not respond quickly to treatment), I

---

[1] 4 grams of aspirin is the generally recommended maximum daily dose for an adult.

decided not to cancel on Sunday but rather to wait until Monday morning. I would take my temperature first thing in the morning. I made a temperature below 37.0 my yardstick – below 37.0, I would head for work, anything from 37 and above and I would not venture outside home!

Lo and behold, on waking up on Monday morning, the thermometer clocked 38.6 degrees Celsius! Not only that, I felt really miserable. Quickly, I switched on my laptop and dispatched an e-mail to my agency to cancel the session for the week.

Without a positive COVID-19 test to base my statement on, I only spoke about flu-like symptoms that had resulted in a fever in my e-mail.

When despite the above measures there was no sign of the condition improving, when the temperature persisted around 38.6 degrees with resultant slight shortness of breath, bitter taste, loss of appetite and feeling so weak as to get out of bed, it dawned on me that I was dealing with something other than common flu.

This was at the time when Europe had become the epicentre of the disease. The media was filled with news of large numbers of deaths in Italy and Spain. As to be expected, I grew a bit scared. I decided therefore to escalate my treatment regime by adding antibiotics.

I want to explain the rationale behind my action. I will do so in in simple terms, for the understanding of the lay person.

In medicine there is a term known as secondary infection or co-infection. In this case I suspected Covid-19, caused by a virus, was the primary infection.

Bacteria tend to take advantage of an ongoing primary infection, in this case Covid-19, to attack the poor victim, to potentially worsen an already bad situation.

Thus, when my condition did not improve despite the measures already touched upon, I said to myself: "Covid on its own is a dangerous 'guy', a potential threat to your life. The hospitals in the UK are already filling up. You cannot afford to allow any bacteria co-infection to worsen your situation!"

So, though it is not standard therapy for one to treat a viral infection with antibiotics, still I decided to take one gram of amoxicillin twice daily as a preventive measure towards averting a possible secondary bacterial infection.

I am sure not every doctor will agree with me on the matter. Well, friend, it was a desperate situation. I did not want this nasty Coronavirus to just emerge from nowhere and send me to my untimely death!

In a hospital setting, I would prescribe according to the standard guidelines. This was, however, my own body, so I had the right to treat myself with the best of intentions.

I kept taking the prophylactic amoxicillin (meant to avert a secondary infection) for a week. Whether it contributed to the favourable outcome, I cannot tell. In any case, I was spared possible pneumonia, a lung inflammation that could have led to a more severe condition, possibly death!

I also resorted to rest. One may not have to spend all the time in bed, but it is very important one avoids straining the body. Sitting in a garden to enjoy fresh air – so long as one is not so weak so to do – could be beneficial.

In all, I battled with the diseases for at least 14 days. Even after the fever had subsided and I began to recover, a weird feeling of burning sensations to the body persisted for several days.

One may want to put me the question: Having survived Covid, what is the impression it has left on you?

I am not an alarmist, but the impression I gained through my own experience is that we are dealing with a disease that plays in a far higher league than common flu.

For example, in the case of the common flu I usually get the temperature under control after a few days. That was not the case with Covid-19. In the case of Covid-19, despite taking 1 gram of paracetamol tablets three to four times daily, the temperature persisted between 37.5 and 38.6 degrees for several days.

Next to mention are the crushing muscle pains, the bitter taste in the mouth, the loss of appetite, feeling generally unwell. I must say that in my case persistent coughing, which is generally associated with the disease, was not a prominent symptom.

I also want to make a comment. It has in the meantime been established that Covid-19 could lead to a blood clot. Indeed, after I had recovered I received the sad news from Germany to the effect that a Ghanaian doctor who I happened to have come across on one occasion when I attended a doctor's seminar had fallen victim to the awful disease. The information I got was that his sad passing was not directly through respiratory failure (which Covid-19 is generally associated with) but rather by way of a stroke.

There is an argument going on within the medical world as to whether Covid-19 patients should routinely be given medication to prevent the development of blood clots. In the hospital setting this would likely be in the form of daily injections.

I mentioned that I started taking aspirin earlier due to my habit of treating common flu that way. Aspirin is generally known for its ability to prevent the building of blood clots. Indeed it is common practice to prescribe low doses of aspirin for those with heart and circulatory problems as well as other underlying medical conditions that make them prone to developing blood clots.

Would the medical world perhaps consider recommending a daily low dose of aspirin (300mg for example) to adults displaying mild to moderate symptoms, who are able to manage their symptoms outside of hospital as a means to prevent the development of blood clots?

Such patients could take 500–1000mg of paracetamol three to four times daily in addition to the aspirin to manage the symptoms of fever, headache and general muscle and bodily aches, just as in my case.

I want the dear reader to consider this as an expressed opinion of a world citizen and not as medical doctor responsible for him or her. If in doubt, the reader should better consult their own doctors.

Though I was certain beyond all doubt that the health scare I had encountered was attributable to the newcomers from Coronaland, for a while I kept it to myself and my nuclear family. I did not want to broadcast the news, not even to other close members of my family without substantiating it.

For a while the tests available on the market were deemed unreliable. After waiting several weeks, two tests, one from an American company and another from a Swiss manufacturer, were generally attested as being almost 100% reliable. At that stage, I paid for a test that made use of one the two testing agents just referred to.

I had indeed reckoned with a positive outcome, and that is exactly how it turned out to be.

Though it is a matter that falls in the realm of medical confidentiality, I have decided to print the report on this page so as to debunk any notion that what I am reporting is invented, something concocted by me to mislead the public.

Notwithstanding the above, I also want to make the following disclaimer. The advice just given is made with the best of intentions, and is based on the general prevailing medical knowledge on the matter of Coronavirus. I am not your doctor, so please do not take it as binding medical advice. If in doubt, please seek the advice of your own doctor.

Name: ROBERT PEPRAH-GYAMFI   **Report Produced by:**

DOB | Age: **X X X X**   **The Doctors Laboratory**

Gender: M

Lab Ref no.: 20T373603
Collected: 26/05/2020 09:00   **Received:**   28/05/2020
11:26LDC HOME VISITS ZONE 1 UNIT 2
PENSBURY STREET LONDON
SW18 4DD
TRACKED24

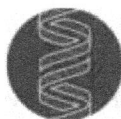

Hospital No.:

Reference:

Report Date: 28 May 2020 16:02:45
IMMUNOLOGY
Anti-SARS CoV 2 IgG Result   POSITIVE
Clinical Comment   SARS-CoV-2 IgG Positive.
Consistent with

SARS-CoV-2 infection at some time. Immunity to re-infection is unknown and must not be assumed. Methodology: ABBOTT CMIA
Please note: This test is CE marked for venesection samples only. Initial samples obtained by self-collection have been verified by the laboratory as performing within the same performance criteria as those taken by venesection and studies are on-going. This test has been submitted to UKAS for accreditation

The End